SILENT RISK

MW00938733

SILENT RISK

Issues about the Human Umbilical Cord

Jason H. Collins, MD, MSCR
Charles L. Collins, MD
Candace C. Collins, MD

To order additional copies of this book, contact:
Xlibris LLC
1-888-795-4274
www.Xlibris.com
Orders@Xlibris.com
128458

CONTENTS

This book is dedicated to the parents who have experienced the loss of a newborn secondary to an umbilical cord accident.

PREFACE

Congenital abnormalities of the human umbilical cord and placenta
may result in significant complications during labour. The ill-effects
are predominantly upon the newborn-less common maternal
morbidity and mortality may result.

—Albert A. Earn, MD, MSc
Winnipeg, Canada 1951

The issue of umbilical cord-related fetal harm and fetal stillbirth is
unaddressed in modern reproductive care. Although observations of
umbilical cord-related deaths have not necessarily proven causation, it
is difficult not to ask, what is the relationship? It is time to answer this
question and to discern the full ramifications of umbilical cord-related
injury and death. The information discussed here is based on twenty-five
years of research and a review of medical journals and texts. The authors
have searched over one thousand peer-reviewed articles published as
of 1950 to provide a current panorama of this reproductive problem,
which is not limited to humans. In addition, the Pregnancy Institute
is dedicated to solving the problem of umbilical cord accidents. The
Pregnancy Institute is a 501(c)(3) nonprofit medical research corporation
cofounded by Jason H. Collins, MD, MSCR, an obstetrician interested
in improving birth outcomes; Charles L. Collins, BSE, MD, a pathologist
interested in placental changes; and Candace C. Collins, MD, a pediatric
ophthalmologist interested in learning disabilities. By assembling this
story, it is our goal to persuade other researchers to turn their attention
to the problem of solving umbilical cord accidents and anomalies.
Hopefully, the future will see a permanent solution. The mother, also, can
play a role in solving the tragedy of umbilical cord accidents. While it is
unknown how much time is needed for a fetus to die, it is believed that
some fetuses die slowly.

Fetal behavior is consistent and can have a repetitive (circadian) rhythm. As discussed later, awareness of fetal movements, sleep-wake cycles, and tendencies may provide an initial warning of a compromised fetus. Verbalizing these changes to the obstetrician may alert everyone of the need for a closer look at the fetus with ultrasound and fetal monitoring. We hope that after reading this book, you, the reader, will have a greater understanding of this tragedy. The expectant mother will hopefully understand her role in solving this tragedy, and the medical professional will realize their responsibility to protect the baby from UCA.

ACKNOWLEDGMENTS

We would like to thank the patients who provided us with the need to find a solution to the problem of umbilical cord accidents. Many parents courageously came forward and shared with us their experiences of umbilical cord-related stillbirth. To discuss these events is difficult for them because to lose a normal fetus is so unique an experience.

Many scientists, researchers, physicians, midwives, and nurses over the years have grappled with this issue. One who stands out in modern times is Jason C. Birnholz, MD, who summarized the issue of the supply line (umbilical cord). In the context of an overall vision he states:

> The practical goal of clinical obstetrics is to deliver an infant who will not only survive but develop without handicap from a prenatal or perinatal insult. (Birnholz 1990)

This goal requires the application of tools called ultrasonography and fetal heart rate monitoring. Because of the efforts of Dr. Douglas Howry and Dr. John J. Wild, we can view the fetus in the uterus. Thanks to Dr. Edward H. Hon, fetal heart rate monitoring became established in obstetrical care. Many individuals have added to these great works and continue to do so today. Now, many differing opinions exist about how effective these tools have been to reproductive care and outcomes. Let there be no mistake—to view the fetus and assess its physiology offers a chance to save a dying fetus where otherwise there would be no chance. Many thanks go to Tulane University Medical Library whose holdings of journals, texts, and special collections offer a repository of knowledge covering two hundred years of obstetrical medicine. Margaret Verzwyvelt, Patsy Copeland, and Cathleen Furlong provided much valuable time retrieving articles and hunting down rare interlibrary loans. Thank you to Mr. W. Postel for allowing the many unusual requests to hold his books at home for weeks. Lastly, thank you to Jeanette Beauman, the executive secretary of the Pregnancy Institute, who typed everything, mailed everything, and did everything to bring this book to reality. Thank you to Patricia Taylor, who donated her editorial expertise and believed in the book.

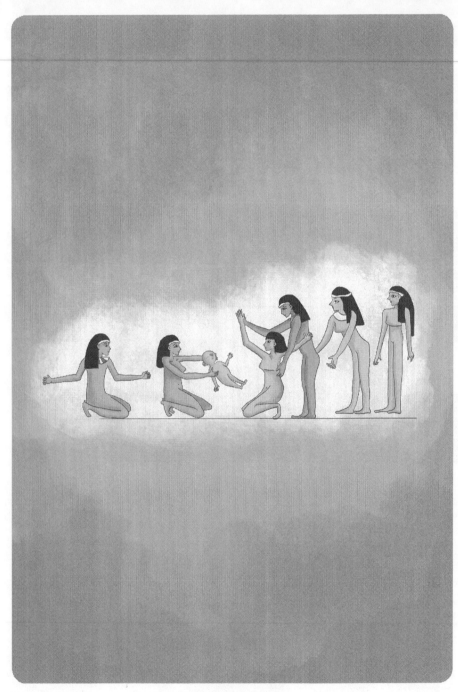

Cleopatra's Birth

INTRODUCTION

A survey of a number of British and American textbooks has yielded scant information on this subject [of umbilical cord complications].
—Kan Pun Shui, BS, MB, and
Nickolson J. Eastman, MD
Hong Kong
1956

It has always been a surprise to me that so little comment has been made on the large proportion of stillbirths which is associated with one or other of the various cord complications.
—T. F. Corkill, MD
Wellington General Hospital
New Zealand
1961

Melbourne Museum has a 375 million year old placoderm fish fossil showing an embryo attached into its mother by an umbilical cord.

One has to wonder what thoughts prehistoric humans had when confronted with the stillbirth of a baby entangled in its umbilical cord.

Egyptian history suggests the placenta with its cord was needed at death to be buried and was kept and stored from birth. Two mummified babies were found in Tutankhamen's tomb and were thought to be stillbirths. No mummified placental or cord remains have been seen.

Some insights from more recent times suggest the umbilical cord represented an omen, a sacred talisman, predictor of future fertility. In Europe, Australia, Africa, and Americas, the umbilical cord was dried and soaked in water for consumption to ensure future fertility. It was eaten, hung from tree branches, and stuffed in volcanic rock crevices at sites such as the Birthing Stones in Kukahiioko, Oahu. In Turkey and Japan, the umbilical cord is preserved. In Japan, there is a special box called *kotobuki bako* in which is preserved a segment of the umbilical cord for future good fortune.

Chinese literature suggests the cord has medicinal properties. European insights beginning with Galen (AD 129-200) suggested the umbilical cord served to nurture the fetus through arteries and veins. Leonardo da Vinci (1452-1519) observed that the cord was as long as the fetus at a given gestational age. Spiglius (1631) determined blood flow direction, and Harvey (1657) suggested that interruption of this blood flow could be the cause of fetal death if the cord was compressed. Early descriptions of fetal loss from cord entanglement date as far back as three hundred years ago.

In 1750, the British obstetrician William Smellie describes case number 172 in his *Treatise on the Theory and Practice of Midwifery* as a stillborn with four cord loops around the neck. One of the first published drawings of an UCA was by Andrew Bell in the *Encyclopedia Britannica* (1769), depicting a fetal death with a combination of one nuchal cord, a body loop, and a true knot (currently on the cover of the Royal College of Obstetricians and Gynaecologists [UK] brochure). By the 1800s, many observations were recorded of distressed fetuses born with cord entanglement and cord abnormalities. UCA was established as a definite cause of stillbirth. Over the last twenty years, images of four cord loops similar to Dr. Smellie's description and management of entangled babies have been peer reviewed and published in medical journals, demonstrating stillbirth can be avoided.

A review of these early descriptions suggest *clinical symptoms* such as pulling sensations felt at the top of the uterus and excessive fetal movement (hyperactivity) followed by decreased fetal activity prior to fetal death. Today, the field of obstetrics is confronted with the issue of umbilical cord complications—a timeless, almost prehistoric example of how imperfect reproductive evolution sometimes can be. Issues of birth-related blood loss, infection, and surgical intervention (C-section) have matured. Premature birth, congenital anomalies, and toxemia still challenge the obstetrical community. Because umbilical cord accidents may represent a small number of fetal deaths, the motivation to

JASON H. COLLINS, MD, MSCR

investigate this reproductive tragedy may not be seen as urgent. However, out of four million births per year in the United States, an estimated eight thousand umbilical cord-related deaths occur. This is known as mortality. What harm occurs to the live-born fetus due to an umbilical cord complication is unknown. Obstetrical scientists call this harm morbidity. This morbidity is studied in terms of delivery outcome—meaning, what harm is noticeable and how much. This harm often goes unnoticed for years. What harm does occur is rarely recorded. Prenatal umbilical cord compression is currently suspected to provide such morbidity as neurologic and cardiac damage and may be as subtle as mild learning disabilities or as obvious as cerebral palsy. This is currently considered speculative by most, but not all, reproductive scientists. The Perinatal Umbilical Cord Project (PUCP), an ongoing project at the Pregnancy Institute, seeks to understand the issue of umbilical cord complications, an event particularly tragic to the mother. If mothers are to be comforted, an explanation of how these events happen is important. The PUCP has established a scientific method (protocol) of observation and has prospectively inspected over one thousand pregnancy cases. Method: All patients receive standard prenatal care starting with an exam at eight to ten weeks. This includes a vaginal ultrasound, a second ultrasound at twenty weeks, and a third ultrasound study at twenty-eight weeks screens for umbilical cord problems. Also, at every visit, the fetal heart rate is studied for ten to fifteen minutes and recorded. Patients identified with umbilical cord abnormalities (UCA) are watched biweekly. Repeat studies with ultrasound and fetal heart rate monitoring occur as needed.

As evidence and data accumulate, the authors hope that a solution can be created that will allow successful management of the normal pregnancy threatened by an umbilical cord complication.

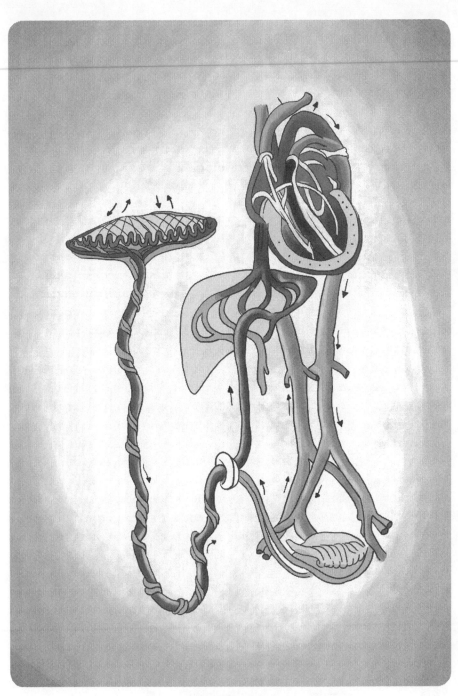

Placental Umbilical Circulation

CHAPTER ONE

Origin and Development of the Umbilical Cord

The human blastocyst implants into uterine decidua . . . There is little realization that this supreme accomplishment is the final stage in several hundred million years of previous, step-by-step preparation of the blastocyst and the uterine mucosa for such a magnificent event.

—Richard Torpin, MD
(Student of the Human Placenta)
Medical College of Georgia
1931-1974

In its extraembryonic site the primitive streak creates a node-like cell reservoir from which the allantois, a universal caudal appendage of all amniotes and the future umbilical cord of placental mammals emerges. This new insight into the fetal/umbilical relationship may explain the etiology of a large number of umbilical-associated birth defects.

—Karen M. Downs
Department of Anatomy
University of Wisconsin-Madison School of Medicine
NIH *Bioessays*
2009

It has been estimated that 30% of births have some type of umbilical cord finding. This statistic implies a potential for fetal harm that may not be appreciated by scientific and public health authorities. Not knowing how many fetuses are harmed by their umbilical cords prevents research into the issue. If neurological harm can occur as the result of umbilical cord problems, then this mechanism of harm to the fetus needs to be investigated. Every fetus should have the opportunity to begin life with all its God-given talents and abilities. Realistically, this may not be possible, but some physically normal newborns could benefit from a reduction in the risks of a cord mishap. It is estimated that learning disabilities may represent 15% of children today. What if one-third of these learning disabilities are due to some type of cord complication? The issue of cerebral palsy is important, but currently, no solution and few insights exist as to its origin. Preventing the stillbirth of a normal infant would be an important step in identifying cord-related harm. What is the size of the problem, and what best describes each part of the problem of umbilical cord mishaps? Disruption of the umbilical cord supply line is a major source of harm to the developing fetus. It is estimated that every third to fourth delivery has an identifiable umbilical cord abnormality or anomaly. What is unknown is how these findings affect the fetus in degrees. The obvious effect is that stillbirth can result from the closing of the supply line.

The Stillbirth Collaborative Research Network recently reported on the probable or possible cause of death of 512 stillbirths whose mothers consented to complete postmortem examination of their baby. Umbilical cord accidents (UCA) were reported to represent 10% of stillbirths. In Caucasians, the UCA-associated stillbirth rate was 13% and 4% in non-Hispanics and blacks. Nine percent of stillbirths were due to hypertension and 8% due to other maternal medical disorders. A literature review places the UCA-associated stillbirth rate at 15%. These databases do not include stillbirth due to several UCA pathologies such as torsion, multiple cord entanglement, and abnormal placental cord insertion. The main reason for these absences is the belief by some that these abnormalities do not cause actual death or recurrent stillbirth. It is now evident that UCA is more important a cause of stillbirth than pregnancy hypertension or gestational diabetes. It is now necessary to develop protocols to identify and manage this problem.

Recommended Reading

The Stillbirth Collaborative Research Network Writing Group, Bukowski, R., M. Carpenter, D. Conway, D. Coustan, D. J. Dudley, R. L. Goldenberg, C. J. Hogue, M. A. Koch, C. B. Parker, H. Pinar, U. M. Reddy, G. R. Saade, R. M. Silver, B. J. Stoll, M. W. Varner, M. Willinger. 2011. "Causes of Death Among Stillbirths." *JAMA* 306 (22): 2459-2468. doi: 10.1001/jama.2011.1823

The umbilical cord is a multidifferentiated organ. Connection to the placenta is one of its many functions. Located at the lower third of the embryo at the primitive ridge, the proximal portion of the umbilical cord begins to form at the allantoic core domain. Between four and six weeks, as the embryonic disc takes a cylindrical shape, the umbilical cord grows and fuses with the placenta. It elongates away from the placenta, forming umbilical cord vessels and increasing in diameter. There are eight different umbilical cord forms, the genetics of which have yet to be studied. The nature of umbilical cord growth may be determined by paternal genes versus the placental genes. The importance of this is, the umbilical cord is not placental in origin and has its own distinct origins. Scientifically it should be treated as a separate organ of reproduction. The proximal fetal attachment is unique and develops a sac (herniation) by ten weeks. This area houses the guts (intestines) until the twelfth week of gestation. At this time, the umbilical cord is short, usually shorter than the head-to-tail (crown-to-rump) length of the embryo and of proportionately large diameter. It is not able to tolerate rotation about itself or the formed embryo. In fact, as the umbilical cord elongates, the proximal cord encompassing the intestinal pouch cannot be disturbed. The distal initial stalk develops in the center of the placental implantation site. The allantois begins at the pole (end) of the embryo and eventually centers itself in the fetus. By twelve weeks, the intestines leave the proximal cord and return to the stomach, the elongation of the cord begins, and the location of the umbilicus (belly button) positions in the middle third of the embryo. The elongation of the umbilical vein and arteries coincides with the development of Wharton's jelly, an umbilical cord connective tissue, the stem cells of which can used for regeneration of various tissues including the heart.

What umbilical cord fundamental factors might contribute to UCA? Different characteristics in umbilical cord structure and function may predispose a given fetus to UCA under stressful conditions. Umbilical cord properties—tensile strength, diameter, circumference, Wharton's jelly content, weight, and length—may be determined genetically. Umbilical cord development, differentiation, growth, and elongation may depend on the sex of the fetus, its nutrition, and well-being. The anatomical connection of the umbilical cord to the fetus and placenta may be independent issues of growth, development, and separation. The human umbilical cord varies in its microstructure, nerves, and elemental content from arteries to vein. Variations in enzyme content of the cord exist from fetus to placenta. There are umbilical cord-vessel cellular and biochemical differences in the umbilical cords of normal and abnormal fetuses. These differences are also noted in vessel response to temperature between vein and artery. As of 2010, there are very few publications on gene expression of the normal placenta and normal cord. Tissue sampling of the placenta and cord may be location based and not uniform. An examination of umbilical cord tissue in smoking mothers reviewed *mRNA* expression. Validation of three *somatomammotropin* genes showed a high correlation between qPCR and microarray expression, suggesting altered gene expression of the fetus. An examination of umbilical cord tissue in bronchopulmonary dysplasia (BPD) babies showed gene expression of the chromatin remodeling pathway. Aberrations of the attachments can affect the function of the umbilical cord. These differences from fetus to fetus may explain the vulnerability of one fetus over another with a similar UCA (such as nuchal cord and as exampled by the 2009 H1N1 swine flu pandemic, which caused deaths in susceptible patients).

Tensile strength: Several reports have measured the breaking point of the human umbilical cord. Because of the differences among cords in Wharton's jelly, collagen content, and muscle layer structure, there is a range of breakage points and sites. The average load required to break the majority of human umbilical cords is 10-14 lb, the range being 4-24 lb (at term, 1.81-10.89 kg). Cords ruptured 22.5% of the time at the placental end (without description of the attachment). Umbilical cord traction forces of 8 lb usually separated the placenta from the uterus. Otherwise, most cord ruptures were within 12 inches of the fetus. The human umbilical cord is elastic and will stretch to 12.5% of its length. The tensile strength may average 2.5% of fetal weight.

As a result, some fetuses may tolerate more traction and loss of slack during entanglement than others. Lastly, *cDNA* microarray analysis of human umbilical vein endothelial cells (HUVECs) under strain point to genetic expression of vasoactive materials and cellular alteration. A condition called mosaicism (more than one pair of genes in the fetus and placenta) has now been reported in the umbilical cord. This suggests that paternal genes may influence cord characteristics more than maternal genes.

Diameter/circumference: The human umbilical cord has a reported average diameter of 1.5 cm and a separately reported average circumference of 3.6 cm after birth. The umbilical vein and artery have been measured before and after birth. The ultrasound average vein diameter is 8 mm with an average artery diameter of 4 mm at term. Various biomechanical characteristics of the umbilical cord such as elasticity, vessel wall thickness, and pressure tolerance have been studied. There is an association with aneuploidy and abnormal diameters.

Umbilical cord cells have a potential to act as multipotential stem cells. These stem cells can transform into anticancer and hematopoietic cells. There may also be potential for anticancer therapy with matrix-derived cells. There are no reported cancers of the umbilical cord.

Length: The human umbilical cord can be totally absent or reach a length of 300 cm. Research has shown that removal of a key area called the allantoic core prior to six weeks disrupts cord substance development. Cord-vessel development can be disrupted by removing key proteins. Umbilical cord length is the only factor associated and documented as a definite risk factor for poor fetal outcome. There is an association of abnormal cord length with neurological abnormalities and low IQ values. A multivariate analysis of a small sample of pregnancies (n = 1087 births) reported an association with long cords and IUGR only. An evaluation of all umbilical cords for extremes of length and development should be considered at all deliveries at this time due to findings in larger studies. There may also be an association with urinary tract abnormalities. There is a tendency for long cords (> 70 cm) to be familial and repeat in the same mother in subsequent pregnancies (Pregnancy Institute data).

Absent or short: Absent or short (< 35 cm) umbilical cords (at 3% of cords) have been described and reported in cases of congenital anomalies. A short cord may be due to reduced fetal activity (such as with twinning—monoamniotic and conjoined). There is a reported association between fetal movement and bone density. This suggests that decreased fetal movement and short cords and low bone density are related. A primary failure of elongation has been noted in association with sirenomelia (lack of adequate fetal blood pressure), schisis, anencephaly (lack of hypothalamic hormones?), acardia (cardiac output?), and adhesions (early amniotic rupture sequence [EARS]). There may be additional molecular factors involved in cord lengthening that are not tension related. Genetic origins may also exist, and placental imprinted genes may play a role in cord length. These limb-body wall complexes (LBWC), although rare, may provide insights into cord development. Placental trisomy 16 is associated with short cord (which may be developmental as a result of restricted fetal movement or directly related to genetic malfunction). Absolutely short cords can interfere with the mechanics of labor and delivery while exhibiting changes in fetal heart rate patterns. This restriction of descent (which is relative to the placental position and insertion) leads to an increase in the incidence of cesarean section, forceps and vacuum extractions. Relatively short cords (lengths compromised by fetal entanglement causing loss of slack) can interfere with delivery as well. As of 2010, there is no published report of a short cord recurrence or familial genetic inheritance. There is one report of prenatal diagnosis of a short cord.

Long umbilical cords: long umbilical cords (> 70 cm at 4% of cords) are documented to be directly associated with poor fetal outcome and associated with UCA, especially fetal entanglement, true knots (sometimes multiple), and torsion. Placental changes are associated with long cords, suggesting blood flow disruption or increased resistance. Male cords are longer than female cords, and term vertex fetuses may have longer lengths than term breech fetuses (with the duration of presentation unknown). Multigravida cord length may be longer than primigravida cord length (the first pregnancy having a shorter length than the third, this may imply more room for movement-tension or more blood supply/hormone production/fetal and maternal weight gain). Twin gestations may have fetuses with discordant lengths and shorter lengths than singletons. Single umbilical artery-vessel structure is increased in long cords. There are no studies considering maternal smoking, alcohol, caffeine, or cocaine ingestion and umbilical cord length in humans (animal studies report shorter cord lengths than controls). Umbilical cord function is not readily impaired by length, and venous return from the placenta to the fetus is maintained regardless of length. There may be an association between viscoelastic behavior of the cord and protection against excessive elongation (which means fetal movement may have a limited effect on cord elongation). There are no studies measuring the umbilical cord prenatally with ultrasound and evaluating the risk factor of cord length for poor fetal outcomes.

Umbilical cord-vessel number: Reports of five vessels, four vessels, fused cords in twins, and two-vessel cords have associated fetal conditions. The best one studied of these findings is umbilical cords with one artery and one vein, single umbilical artery (SUA).

Single umbilical artery (SUA) cases have been reported with a variety of genetic, anomalous, and stillbirth outcomes. There are SUA findings associated with trisomy malformations but no confirmed genetic sequence associations with UCA to date. SUA is considered to be a developmental UCA associated with disturbance of fetal blood flow. There are two forms of SUA: a helical form and a straight form. Many observations have been published about this umbilical cord maldevelopment that is seen at 7% of abortus up to twenty-eight weeks, at 7% twins, and occurs at 1% of term pregnancies. There may be an association between the left or right umbilical artery that is absent and increased risk of fetal abnormalities. There may be several categories of SUA depending on which vessel represents the umbilical artery (vitelline, allantoic, R or L umbilical). There is also a difference in malformations depending on whether the right or left vein persists. SUA is associated with stillbirth with an incidence of 3%-20%. SUA is common in twins and diabetic pregnancies, in association with long cords and small placentas. Finding an SUA on ultrasound screening should place the pregnancy on alert for associated developments. Trisomies, especially those with mosaic genetics, should be reviewed for fetal anomalies. A finding of SUA entanglement or decreased fetal weight should prompt closer fetal evaluation.

Umbilical cord-vessel morphology may be a risk factor for the fetus. The normal umbilical cord may have been best illustrated and described in 1882 by E. S. Tarnier: an arterial pair mildly helical around a straight vein (with helical muscle bundles by microscopy). Umbilical cord morphology (design) is established by ten to twelve weeks. The normal umbilical cord has six to eight embedded helixes. These helixes do not unwind, are 360 degrees, and cannot be untwisted. The term *helixes* is the proper nomenclature (not *coils, curls, turns, spirals, chirals,* or *twists*). Umbilical cord helixes are fundamental to umbilical cord development and normal function. Other morphologies should be considered abnormal. There are differences in umbilical cord shape that may predispose the fetus to UCA. There may be eight different types (forms) of umbilical cords. There are biochemical differences within the umbilical cord from placenta to fetus that are distinct in compromised fetuses versus normal fetuses. It is theorized that several factors may determine umbilical cord shape. Fetal cardiac output, predominance of umbilical artery blood flow, and fetal symmetry may be important. Study by Doppler velocimetry of cord length, artery pairs, and helical types have suggested some differences that may be important, but fetal outcomes were not always reported. There may be an inherent role of the umbilical cord to assist the fetal heart. If so, umbilical cord morphology may change this assist action or "pulsometer." Thrombosis of the umbilical vein may disrupt this pump-assist action and lead to stillbirth. Previous studies on UCA have not fully considered the differences that may be inherent in these different forms.

Umbilical cord attachments: There is specialized anatomy for the umbilical cord attachment to the placenta and fetus. Failure of these attachments will cause fetal death. The umbilical ring is designed to allow for fetal growth without umbilical cord detachment until delivery. The umbilical ring is innervated, and these nerves have branches that connect to the vagus trunks and phrenic nerves. There are connecting branches to the right adrenal gland and maybe to the proximal umbilical cord. This neuronal pattern may suggest an umbilical ring to the ductus venosus feedback system, which partly regulates blood flow to the fetal cardiovascular system. Failure of proper umbilical cord development at the fetal attachment can cause stillbirth. As stated previously, absent umbilical cord syndrome is fatal. Other defects can be due to embryonic structures and remnants at the proximal cord. Proximal umbilical cysts, urachal anomalies, and vitelline-vessel anomalies have been well described in pathology texts. Periumbilical skin length may also have extremes, of which long skin lengths have been noted in dysmorphic children and UCA in horses. Velamentous insertion (VI) comes in various forms. It is an abnormal attachment to the membranes instead of the placenta. Its impact on the fetus is dependent on placental position (360 degrees in the uterus and insertion direction dependent). Velamentous insertion over the uterine cervix is called vasa previa. It is now possible to identify VI by multiple methods: ultrasound, color Doppler, 3-D imaging, which includes MRI. The prenatal diagnosis of VI is now a requirement of twenty-first-century obstetrical practice. Once diagnosed, this UCA can be managed, and stillbirth can be prevented. VI can be visualized by the eighteen-week to twenty-week ultrasound.

Recommended Reading Risk Factors and Outcomes of Velamentous and Marginal Cord Insertions; A population-based study of 634,741 pregnancies: Cebbing, T Kiserud, S Johnson, S Albrichtsen PLOS; July 2013 Volume 8

The responsibilities of the cord are numerous. For example, the cord manages its own growth, elongation, and expansion; accommodates increasing blood flow; and possibly assists the fetal heart. It also must regulate blood flow and its fluidity (thickness/thinness). In addition, the umbilical arteries and vein contain muscular coats that allow constriction of the vessels at birth or dilation of the vessels during growth. The umbilical cord also must produce its own chemistry to prepare for its role in birth and separation from the newborn umbilicus (a process which takes seven to ten days). Located within the cord are the umbilical vein and arteries. The relationship of the umbilical vein to the umbilical arteries changes with development. These changes can result in cord abnormalities, which will be discussed in the next chapter. Initially, two arteries send blood with waste products from the embryo to the afterbirth (placenta), and the one umbilical vein sends oxygen and nutrient-enriched blood to the embryo from the placenta. This circulation pattern must respond over time to the constantly changing fetal requirements and demands.

Rare developmental changes, which can occur to the embryonic umbilical cord, are persistent of the right vitelline vein, creating a four-vessel cord with two arteries and two veins. The reverse of this is obliteration of an artery and vein and the development of a two-vessel cord with one artery and one vein. There also exists a description of a double cord within separate vessel duplication. Genetic problems are seen with two-vessel cords where fetuses with multiple malformations have defective organs that are not compatible with life. Maldevelopment of the genitourinary system such as bladder and kidney has been noticed. Although these relationships are known, obstetrics currently does not place any added concern on pregnancies with two-vessel cords. No remedy for these anomalies presently exists. Umbilical cord vessels may multiply and branch under stressful conditions. For example, heavy smoking is associated with multiple channels in the umbilical cord. Hypoxia (the decrease of available oxygen) has been determined as the stimulus for opening of early vestigial vessels of the cord, once closed at ten weeks. These findings of rechanneled embryonic vessels are also associated with fetal compromise and stillbirths. A trend was also noted in which first-time pregnancies had more vascular branching than multiple-birth mothers. Research indicates a 2% probability of this cord finding. How the umbilical cord elongates and grows is unknown. As it grows, it changes the relationship between the vein and arteries. These changes may or may not predispose the growing fetus to blood flow disturbances or mechanical disturbances between the fetus and umbilical cord. The umbilical cord is traditionally thought to stretch or elongate depending on the activity of the fetus. Active fetuses are believed to have longer cords on the whole than less active fetuses. Twins and triplets, because of restricted movement, have been shown to have cords, on the average, shorter than their single counterparts. Boys have longer cords than girls. Nonidentical twins have varying cord lengths when compared to each other. Nonidentical twin A can have a cord twice the length of twin B. Also, twins A and B can have different cord architectures where one is straight and one is helical.

Rare instances exist in which no cord develops at all, the fetus being attached directly to the placenta at the umbilicus. Other reports in Chinese and French literature cite cords as long as 300 cm in length. The umbilical cord appears to have organ-like properties. These properties are prone to disturbance under certain conditions that can affect the fetus.

Just as a heart can fail pumping or the liver and kidney can fail filtering the body's chemistry and waste products, the umbilical cord can fail in its role of being a supply line.

Wharton's Jelly

Wharton's jelly is a specialized tissue serving many purposes for the developing fetus. Its specialized cells contain gelatin-like mucus that encases fibers. These properties give it an elastic and cushiony effect, which can tolerate the vibration, bending, stretching, and twisting of an active fetus. In addition, it holds the vessels together, may regulate blood flow, plays a role in providing nutrition to the fetus, stores chemistry for the onset of labor, and protects the supply line. Umbilical cords without much Wharton's jelly are more prone to compression, and complete absence is usually associated with fetal death. If an umbilical cord is twisted or knotted, it is more likely to tighten where there is less resistance, such as an area low in Wharton's jelly. It is believed that males have more Wharton's jelly content than do females and that good nutrition increases the amount. Wharton's jelly tends to reduce with gestational age and can disappear when pregnancies go beyond forty weeks. Because these cases tend to have fetal heart rate changes, the level of Wharton's jelly is a consideration when obstetricians plan the deliveries of pregnancies low on amniotic fluid.

Cord Length

Cord length can be associated with neurologic abnormalities and fetal positioning. To understand this correlation, it is important to understand the physiology of the human umbilical cord. Cord length has been frequently measured. One of the largest studies was completed by pathologist Dr. Richard Naeye. In his book *Disorders of the Placenta, Fetus, and Neonate*, Dr. Naeye averages the lengths of different umbilical cords at progressively older gestational ages. The cord is believed to elongate until as late as thirty-six weeks although rapid change occurs until twenty-eight weeks then slows. The final length of the umbilical cord averages about 61 cm, or 24 inches, according to Percy Malpas, MD, a British obstetrician who studied cord length in the 1960s.

The first pregnancy tends to generate a shorter cord than subsequent pregnancies. Although no published report of a genetic relationship exists, there may be one. So why 61 cm? Umbilical cords of whales, porpoises, goats, and other mammals are relatively shorter than the human cord. Walker and Rye of Cambridge surmised in the *British Medical Journal* in 1960 that prehistoric humans evolved length for protection. Nature's purpose was to allow the mother to pick up the newborn without disturbing the placenta. The event of breast feeding would then separate the placenta—an event which could attract predators. Having the fetus in tow would allow escape for mother and child.

Today, cord length correlates to several outcomes. Cords too short and cords too long predispose the fetus to intrauterine dangers. A short cord has a length of less than 32 cm. This length was determined in 1910 by a famed Chicago obstetrician, Dr. Joseph B. DeLee. Dr. DeLee believes 32 cm to be the minimal length necessary for a term fetus to deliver. The concept changes, however, when cord insertion site and cord entanglement are considered. This idea is called a relatively short cord. Very short cords less than 20 cm are associated with genetic malformations. When cord lengths were evaluated for IQ, short cords showed a higher incidence of neurologic abnormalities. Cord length may also influence fetal position. Torgrim Sørnes, MD, a Norwegian researcher, observed this. His work suggests that breech-positioned fetuses have shorter cords due to less activity. This insight suggests that if the fetus persists at remaining breech, a cord etiology should be considered, and the obstetrician should watch for fetal difficulties during labor. Umbilical cord circumference and diameter are also important measurements. On average, normal umbilical cords are 3.7 cm in circumference with a range of 3-5 cm. The diameter range of 1.0 cm to 3.0 cm can suggest an abnormal cord with edema, tumor, or hernia. Dimensions greater than a 6 cm circumference should prompt an examination of the cord and fetus. Are shorter cords thicker than longer cords? Although rarely published, it appears that this may be the case. Before cutting any thick cord, it should be checked to ensure that the fetal intestine is not present within the cord. Growth and development of the umbilical cord are dependent upon many factors. Disturbance of these events can lead to fetal compromise or result in fetal compromise. These effects will be described in the next chapter.

Umbilical Cord Design

How the umbilical cord is built has long been of interest to anatomists. A look at all mammals shows a variety of design adaptations. In humans, it has been determined that there are several designs. What these differences mean to the fetus is unknown. Attempts by several noted scientists to understand how the umbilical cord works have taught us that the cord is more like an organ rather than a rigid conduit (pipeline).

Not all cords are alike. Just as there are different kinds of hair (curly/straight, thick/thin), there are different kinds of cords. Most cords (99%) have three vessels although some (1%) have only two, and even less have four. The relationship between the normal vein and two arteries is usually parallel (figure 7). This parallel configuration can vary, however, and may imply effects that can alter blood supply to the fetus. Variances include arteries that are together or separated with each artery lateral to the vein (figure 8). Another variance is arteries that wind around the vein while the vein remains central in the cord. This is sometimes referred to as spiraled arteries, but *helical* is the preferred term (figure 9). The vein can also parallel the arteries in a helical configuration, and the vein can wind around the arteries. Several researchers have concentrated on these differences and suggest that umbilical cords of absolutely straight designs may be more prone to disruptions of blood flow. If these observations are verified, it may be important to know the cord design prior to delivery. The location of umbilical cord attachment to the fetus and placenta is also important. Placental attachments can be in the center, off-center, on the edge, or in the membranes. Membranous insertions of the umbilical cord are called velamentous insertions. These placental cord designs have flaws that can lead to cord tears. Currently, little research has been done to develop prenatal diagnostic criteria. Umbilical attachment of the cord can vary and predispose the infant to hernias at the umbilicus and constriction of the cord. Although these are uncommon findings, future research will allow a more accurate evaluation of the umbilicus. Amniotic bands can interfere with both ends of the umbilical cord. For example, the amniotic membrane can leave remnants in the form of fibrous bands, which can stiffen and occlude the blood circulation through the cord.

These events are reproductive mishaps that have no current remedy. In order to begin the process of creating solutions to umbilical cord-related complications, understanding cord function and design must be thorough.

Umbilical Cord Abnormalities and Anomalies

Throughout human history, stillbirths have been associated with umbilical cord findings. These findings vary, and some are more common than others.

Scientifically, umbilical cord changes and effects are described several ways. To start, the umbilical cord can develop design flaws that can lead to fetal harm. These flaws are called umbilical cord abnormalities:

Table 1	
Short Cords	less than 35 cm
Long Cords	more than 70 cm
Two-Vessel Cords	one artery/one vein
Four-Vessel Cords	two arteries/two veins
Velamentous Insertions	inserted on the membranes
Marginal Insertions	inserted on the placental edge
Constriction of the Umbilicus	lack of Wharton's jelly at the fetal insertion
Wharton's jelly cysts	mucinous Myxoid Edema Growths and Cysts of the Umbilical Cord Umbilical Artery Angioma/Aneurysm Umbilical Vein Varices/ False Knots Hematoma/Teratoma/Thrombosis/Rupture

These abnormal umbilical cords are predisposed to rupture, mechanical failure, entanglement, disruption of labor, uterine malfunction, and premature labor. The ultimate effects are disturbance of the lifeline and derangement of blood flow to the fetus. The difficulty lies in the fact that these abnormalities are silent and invisible. Short umbilical cords (less than 35 cm) are predisposed to rupture and prevention of fetal descent during labor. Very short cords, less than 25 cm, are associated with genetic malformations. Short umbilical cords need to be considered

JASON H. COLLINS, MD, MSCR

relative to their attachments to the placenta. The further the attachment is from the cervix, the less likely the fetus can be born vaginally, requiring a C-section. In addition, fetal heart rate changes will be more likely to occur during monitoring, creating concern for all involved in the labor process. Very short umbilical cords, less than 25 cm, have been associated with neurologic disorders, IQs less than 80, and cerebral palsy. There is an increase in stillbirth risk with short and relatively short cords. This risk may be as much as six times more likely, especially when other factors like toxemia are involved. Short cords and cigarette smoking tend to result in small babies, called IUGR (intrauterine growth retarded). It is difficult to unravel the relationships mentioned above since some fetuses may incur neurologic damage, which predisposes them to decreased activity and leads to decreased cord length. Long umbilical cords (longer than 70 cm) are associated with a number of circumstances that can impact fetal life. Leonardo da Vinci studied cord length and believed it was a proportional/natural relationship of 1 to 1 (cord length = fetal age in weeks). Although this is not precisely correct, da Vinci was correct in that it is proportional. Biological and physical principles that dictate the shape of a starfish, tree leaf, or nautilus shell determine the positive or negative relationship between the fetus and its umbilical cord (and probably placenta). Fetal activity is believed to determine umbilical cord growth. This mechanical stimulus may be a direct or indirect factor. How does the umbilical cord grow and elongate? Biochemical and cellular mechanisms must be at work. All these molecular genetic pieces are potentially at risk for failure by inside or outside disturbances. Growth factors have been identified in the umbilical cord. In addition, studies in twins suggest a genetic control or modulation of length. Length can also be influenced by amniotic fluid volume and anything that constricts fetal movement. Umbilical cords are also innervated to a degree near the umbilicus. The role this plays or whether there is an influence on cord development is currently unknown. Of all those multiple variables influencing cord length, the most important variable needs to be determined. It is unknown whether individual cell enlargement or cell division and multiplication cause cord growth. Many different cells such as muscle cells, endothelial cells, fibroblasts, connective cells, and amniotic cells must all do the same thing. Insight into this aspect of fetal development may help understand anomalies of the cord. Microscopic comparison of long and short cords may reveal differences of structure. Thickness or thinness of vessel walls, composition of Wharton's jelly, and artery-vein interrelationships may be important findings that explain long-cord susceptibility to various events. Two-vessel cords occur in about 1% of births. The connection to fetal harm or well-being is unclear. These umbilical cords have one artery and one vein. The dominant artery origination (left or right inside the fetus) determines whether or not congenital malformations may be present. It is accepted that these cords may predispose the fetus to stillbirth compared to a normal three-vessel cord. The risk of stillbirth can be six times greater than normal, especially when other factors such as toxemia exist. Whether or not other variables are involved remains to be determined. Development of a single umbilical artery cord may be associated with maternal smoking, drug exposure, placental abnormalities, and maternal diabetes. Whether or not all infants with a two-vessel cord are predisposed to some difficulty remains to be seen. The mechanism of how one artery is obliterated versus undeveloped may be important to understanding this issue. Four-vessel umbilical cords are rare and are mentioned to emphasize the vulnerability of cord vessels to malformation. Not all umbilical cords are alike, and nonidentical twins can have nonidentical cords. Proper development of the embryo and its supply line is an important step toward a healthy fetus and newborn. Maldevelopment of the supply line from the start can predispose the fetus to harm. Another important step in umbilical cord development is the connection of the fetus and placenta to each other. The fetal connection is specialized and has a specific architecture. This design needs to function as a secure tether for the fetus, as a disrupter for umbilical separation (in mammals, the cord tears free or is chewed free), and perhaps, as a sensor for blood flow into the fetus, and must merge with the skin. Researchers have identified nerve endings near the umbilical insertion of the cord in the Wharton's jelly. These end nests may play a role in communicating with fetal valves, called shunts, relative to blood volume-wave properties entering the fetal circulation through the umbilical vein at the level of the liver and heart. When the umbilical end is malformed, constriction or coarctation occurs, stopping blood flow. How this happens is unknown. At the other end of the supply line, the fetal arteries enter the placenta with a membranous support tether and distribute in a branching manner. When the placenta develops, it sometimes migrates and dissolves from its original site. This sometimes can result in what appears to be a relocation of the placenta. The placenta tissue dissolves, leaving a membrane (the amnion), which can then be the connection (insertion) site of the umbilical cord. This

JASON H. COLLINS, MD, MSCR

results in the umbilical cord placental end looking like it is connected to the edge of the placenta (called a marginal or battledore insertion) and a membranous insertion called a (velamentous) insertion. Another variation is called a furcate cord insertion in which the cord does not connect to the placenta, but its branching elements do; however, no membranous insertion exists. These malformations account for another 0.5% to 1% of all births and are observed to increase in premature labor, premature birth, fetal stillbirth, and neurologic harm.

The risk of cord-vessel rupture is increased with an abnormal cord insertion. The difficulty of managing an incident such as cord rupture is great. What makes the mystery even more complicated is the location of the cord insertion in the uterus. If the membranous insertion is over the cervical opening, the risk of tearing and fetal blood loss is great. If a marginal insertion is against the sacrum (lower backbone), the risk of compression and fetal circulation disruption is great as the fetus descends into the pelvis. This relationship of vessel location to fetal location has caused sudden fetal distress and the need to activate a surgical team for an emergency C-section. It is unknown how often this happens during day-to-day obstetrical care as the attention is on the fetus, not the placenta, its location, or its cord-insertion architecture. Umbilical cords may have eight different types of design. The extremes are very helical cords (95%) and completely straight cords (5%). The association between umbilical vein and arteries can vary where veins wind around arteries, veins and arteries are parallel, and arteries wind around veins. The veins can be parallel with the arteries as well (10%). Very helical designs (spiraled, coiled, and curled) may predispose the fetus to certain blood flow changes, and very straight designs may be susceptible to compression. It is unknown what the fetal effects are, but some evidence points to supply-line vulnerability when the design is faulty. Add to this other variables such as placental location and umbilical cord insertion site and the combination becomes a significant factor in determining the well-being of the fetus. Knowing these details may provide important insights into the development of fetal harm. Wharton's jelly, although apparently inert looking, may be an important chemical factory for the fetus. Additionally, its components and cellular makeup can predispose the fetus to the formation of tumors, cysts, and edema. Edema is not an infrequent finding at delivery of a newborn (10%). It is usually limited to small sections of the umbilical cord and associated with trauma due to fetal behavior. Extensive involvement of the cord is associated with complications of pregnancy such as toxemia and infections. When cause is due to fetal circulatory disturbances, fetal heart failure may predispose the cord to edema, which is associated with an increased risk of stillbirth. Tumors can develop in Wharton's jelly. Although rare, teratomas have been reported. Teratomas grow to large sizes and can disrupt vessels and blood flow. Embryonic features of the umbilical cord can produce six types of remnants, some of which look like hemangiomas, blood vessels which, together, look like small varicose veins in a bundle. Other structures such as vitelline duct remnants and urachal duct remnants can be seen. Those changes are very infrequent but should be considered if an enlargement or localized mass is seen in the cord. Hematomas (bleeds into the substance of the cord) can occur and mimic these rare tumors. The possible association with fetal defects must always be considered. As the fetus ages, it is believed that Wharton's jelly recedes. This becomes an important issue when deciding to deliver a postdate infant, where the due date has been passed without delivery. Loss of Wharton's jelly may put the fetus at risk of cord compression and, therefore, fetal harm.

Growths and Swellings of Umbilical Cord Vessels

Like any vessel in the human adult body, umbilical cord vessels can develop sacs, protrusions, bulges, and varicosities. For example, cord vessels can protrude and thrombose like varicose veins or hemorrhoidal veins. In addition, the umbilical vein sometimes bunches up on itself, creating the appearance of a false knot or of multiple varicosities; these spaces can act like quiet pools of blood that can clot and predispose the fetus to a thromboembolism. The clot can break free and enter the fetal circulation or can obstruct cord blood flow. The umbilical arteries can develop similar pockets called aneurysms. These bulges in the arterial vessel wall can rupture and lead to fetal hemorrhages in the uterus. These alterations of structure can predispose the cord to rupture as well. Human umbilical arteries consist of two layers of muscle fibers, the outer layer being three-fourths of the wall thickness and an inner layer. The design of the muscle cells is parallel, where the inner layer runs with the vessel lengthwise and the outer layer surrounds the vessel like a spiral staircase. A thin layer of cells lines the vessel opening, and an outer layer is formed by connective tissue and Wharton's jelly. This architecture allows constriction and shortening of the vessel. Defects in this structure can occur that may predispose the umbilical arteries to failure. A type of architectural defect is called umbilical cord-vessel segmental thinning. In this malformation (1%), umbilical vessel walls are missing a layer of muscle, therefore weakening the vessel. Related observations include fetal anomalies and perinatal problems. These fetuses are predisposed to stillbirth, meconium, and fetal heart rate decelerations. All in all, when a combination of defects results, the risk of umbilical cord failure begins to become important. It is unknown how many placentas and umbilical cords contain a variety of architectural anomalies or abnormalities that lead to miscarriage. It is unknown how much fetal harm may be the result of faulty placentation and cord alterations, such as straight cord segments resulting from the molding of Wharton's jelly due to long-term compression of an entangled cord.

Future research into these issues will be both exciting and fruitful. The integration of the anatomy (structure), biochemistry (substance), and physiology (function) of the umbilical cord will allow the emergence of a new awareness of three structures to manage in pregnancy: the placenta, umbilical cord, and fetal unit.

How the Human Umbilical Cord Works (Physiology)

What is remarkable about the umbilical cord is that it is a blood vessel without branches. This is unique compared to the large blood vessels of the adult body—the aorta and vena cava. Its properties, therefore, are different in some respects and alike in others. The umbilical cord has two-way traffic: the arteries carry blood pumped by the heart away from the fetus, and this circulation surrounds the vein normally; the umbilical vein returns blood to the fetus from the placenta rejuvenated with oxygen and nutrients and devoid of waste products. How this happens is still surrounded by mystery. The fetal heart cannot expand or work harder because it is surrounded by a fluid-filled lung, like pushing against a water bed. Therefore, as the fetus steadily grows exponentially and three-dimensionally, how does it accommodate the increased blood volume it needs over time? As the fetus grows, the cord elongates and grows in diameter. The fetus has to work against a larger column of fluid and tissue resistance at the placental end. It has been estimated that by thirty-one weeks, the umbilical cord must carry seventy quarts of blood per day, moving at four miles an hour. This remarkable organ also must participate in fetal growth milestones; additionally, it may act as an assist pump to the fetal heart. This assist pump may be designed to help the fetus over difficult growth proportions that may exist at twenty weeks, twenty-four weeks, twenty-eight weeks, and thirty-two weeks—times that are known for premature labor to appear. The extra stress on the fetus may require that the cord be designed correctly so that it can have properties of an assist mechanism or pump. This theory, proposed in the 1950s, requires that the arteries surround the vein in the proper architecture. If this is so, then future research into this issue may explain fetal effects secondary to cord design. To date, no assist-pump property has been detected in the umbilical cord. How blood flow is regulated in addition to being carried by the umbilical cord is unclear.

Cord length does not significantly affect blood flow dynamics; however, blood flow must meet some resistance for the circulation to work. As a result, the umbilical arteries are surrounded with four layers of smooth muscle to maintain a certain amount of muscular tone. The umbilical vein is not as muscled. The system operates fully dilated, but stimuli from chemistry or hormones can affect the system and cause constriction. This must happen at birth to reduce blood loss. In larger mammals, the cord must constrict from the placenta to the fetus for the fetus to avoid anemia. In the human, similar mechanisms may be available chemically. Regulation of blood flow, vessel constriction at birth, and blood-loss prevention may be the roles of these vessel-active substances. Some of these substances originate in the placenta. Researchers using ultrasonography recently have been able to measure umbilical blood flow with color Doppler imaging. This technique allows visualization of the blood vessels based on the movement of the blood itself. These studies also suggest that the umbilical vein, arteries, and placenta act as assist pumps of sorts to the fetal heart. Measurement of blood flow allows the obstetrician to determine whether enough blood volume is circulating in the placenta to provide nutrition and oxygen to the fetus. Under certain conditions, this blood flow can be reduced and circulation in the placenta altered to create a growth-affected fetus, intrauterine growth retardation (IUGR). In essence, it is a way of determining the fetus's blood pressure. These findings become important because, in addition to the potential for fetal harm or stillbirth, important lifetime tendencies are emerging.

JASON H. COLLINS, MD, MSCR

The fetus seems to have the ability to set its vital signs for its adult life. If stressed, the IUGR fetus sets blood pressure and heart function, which can predispose the fetus to adult heart attack. These mechanisms are just beginning to be understood, and the umbilical cord may be an important part of the mystery.

A case of a term stillbirth with a straight umbilical cord design with an abnormal placenta, a marginal umbilical cord insertion, and a double nuchal cord was reported from Paris, France, in 1893.

UMBILICAL CORD LESIONS

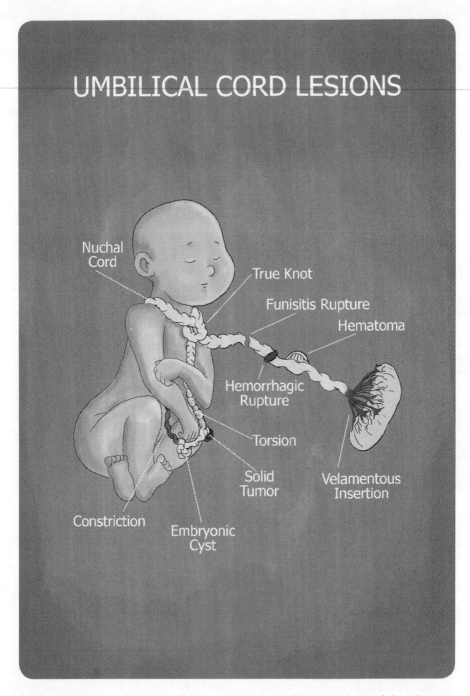

Heifetz, S. A. "Pathology of the umbilical cord." *Pathology of the Placenta.* 2nd edition. Edited by S. H. Lewis and E. Perrin. NY, NY: Churchill Livingstone.

CHAPTER TWO

The Umbilical Cord: The Problems of Supply and Demand

For the layman and more so to the obstetrician, [the umbilical cord] presents a potential hazard during delivery. It is highly desirable that umbilical cords should be examined at delivery.

—Bholanath B. Nadkarni
Professor of Pathology
University of Ottawa/Ontario
Canada, 1969

Many pathologic features of the umbilical cord affect fetal well-being adversely.

—Kurt Benirschke, MD
Professor Emeritus
Department of Pathology University Medical Center
San Diego, California, 1994

Disruption of the umbilical cord (the fetal supply line) may be a source of harm to the developing fetus. An estimated 30% of pregnancies carried to term have some type of umbilical placental abnormality. This means that every third to fourth delivery has an identifiable umbilical cord abnormality or anomaly. What is unknown is how these findings affect the fetus and to what degree. This chapter discusses the types of umbilical cords and their potential inherent complications. The obvious unwanted effect of supply-line disruption is stillbirth. The most dramatic example of this obstruction is an emergency called prolapsed umbilical cord. Prolapse of the cord occurs when a fetus is not properly positioned in the pelvis. Membranes rupture and wash the cord out of the cervix in front of the fetal buttock or head. When the fetal body engages the cervix, the cord is compressed, and blood flow to the fetus ceases. If the patient has the good fortune of being near an operating room, the fetus has ten minutes before harm begins. If a C-section can be performed quickly enough, the infant usually survives without harm. Many variations of this event exist in which factors such as time, degree of compression, and age of the fetus play a role. Yet the common thread among these variations is immediate danger to the fetus. Compression of the umbilical cord obstructs blood flow to and from the fetus. This total obstruction denies the fetus oxygen and blood flow pressure, and it releases stress factors from endocrine organs that contribute to fetal harm.

Umbilical cord compression clearly plays a role in disturbing the well-being of the fetus. The effects of incomplete cord compression are unknown. These impacts are altered by different effects at different gestational ages under various conditions at varying intervals. Current obstetrics continues to debate these issues. Although stillbirth clearly can be caused by a variety of mechanisms creating cord compression, prolapse of the umbilical cord is the only witnessed event that is acknowledged and accepted as a fatal cause-effect complication. The chance of having a prolapsed cord at birth is 1 out of 239 cases to 1 out of 865 cases. The reported chance of fetal loss from a prolapsed cord is 8.6% to 49% of these prolapse occurrences. Similar mechanisms can occur inside the uterus with the same results. One such occurrence is that it can take place with monoamniotic twins. These twins have no barrier between them and can entangle their cords. Stillbirths often occur in one twin or both because of knots and encirclement. It is accepted that these mechanisms do cause stillbirth. On the basis of this knowledge, examination and anticipation of other cord complications are not difficult (table 1). Obstetrical thought now accepts that monoamniotic twins can interfere with each other's umbilical cord. Pregnancies of monoamniotic twins showing no other risk factors or complications are monitored carefully for this supply-line disruption. Published case reports have been described of entangled twins with multiple knots. Intensive surveillance

JASON H. COLLINS, MD, MSCR

was needed for these monoamniotic twins. These reports have described early intervention when fetal heart rate changes suggested the need for delivery as early as thirty-one weeks. If this concept is recognized for monoamniotic twins, why is it not recognized for single fetuses with cord anomalies or abnormalities?

Table 1
Worldwide frequency (incidence) of umbilical cord events and stillbirths (mortality)
To date, a world literature review suggests the following:
U C A Incidence Mortality
Single umbilical artery .2%-3.6% 7%
Non-coiled cords 4.3% Unknown
True Knots 1% 6%
Nuchal Cords 14%-30% Unknown
Body Loops 1% 10%
Short Cords Unknown Unknown
Velamentous Cords .54%-2%, 17% 30%
Torsional cords 6% 20%

Regardless of mechanisms such as prolapsed cord or twins, the pathophysiology is the same: supply line deprivation, restriction of blood flow, and reduction of oxygen and nutrients to the fetus to the degree that injury or death can occur. What does such a mechanism look like? Again, 30% of fetuses delivered have some finding. What are the varied types of cord abnormalities and accidents that can affect the fetus? Some observations from history give us clues. Leonardo da Vinci was not only an artist but also a sculptor and engineer. He recognized in the human form the same principles of proportion as seen in nature. The Greeks had defined many proportions and believed them keys to understanding life. The fetus is proportioned to itself. The early fetus is seen in thirds and the growing fetus in fourths. The term fetus can be seen in fifths, and it can develop entanglement once the umbilical cord is proportionally long. This seems to suggest the point at which the cord begins to pose a danger. This point begins with the cord being four-fifths as long as the fetal head-to-toe length. At this length, the neck can be encircled 360 degrees. This can often happen after ten to twelve weeks' gestational age. A cord of lesser proportional length can't completely encircle the neck. Cord length plays a role in how a fetus develops, how labor is tolerated, and how delivery occurs. What are the different cord-length effects that have been reported in the medical literature?

Absent umbilical cords: If the umbilical cord does not develop, the fetus can develop but can be malformed. The fetus is directly attached to the placenta at the abdomen and usually develops defects. Fetuses without cords have been born by C-section. Without an umbilical cord, life is usually not possible. Yet this concept was not always apparent. The roles played by the placenta, cord, and fetal heart were not realized until the late 1700s.

Short umbilical cords: A cord can be short (20 cm) but can allow delivery if it is attached to the placenta near the cervix. Yet, as previously described, short umbilical cords can affect the fetus. Restriction of movement may occur for genetic or other reasons. Fetal movements may predispose the cord to compression, constriction, and during labor, failure to progress through the birth canal. Short cords can also be responsible for fetal distress during labor, separation of the placenta, and rupture of the umbilical cord prenatally or during labor. In addition, short cords can predispose the umbilical vein and arteries to tears, which can lead to hematomas (vessel rupture) of the cord. Inversion of the uterus (inside out and a medical emergency) can occur from traction on a short cord. Dr. Smellie describes a case of this type. A relatively short cord is a cord that is entangled with the fetus. Although the length is normal, it is caught over the shoulder or around the arm or neck and uses up slack, becoming mechanically unable to allow vaginal delivery. Disruption, compression, and rupture of the cord can occur in a cord that is relatively short. Prenatally addressing a condition of this type will be discussed in chapter 5.

Long umbilical cords: As previously described, a long cord would be considered greater than 70 cm although 90 cm has been used as the measurement. Perhaps a long cord in an abnormal sense should be defined as the length of cord that can cause fetal harm by entanglement. If so, such a cord would be four-fifths as long as the fetus. Long cords become a problem when circumstances predispose the cord to prolapse (slip out of the womb) and are more likely to prolapse simply because there is more of it. In addition, the umbilical cord is heavier than amniotic fluid and therefore sinks. When visualizing the cord with

JASON H. COLLINS, MD, MSCR

ultrasound, a cord may seem suspended in the amniotic fluid because of hydrostatic pressure and position. It may appear to float at the top of the uterus, depending on the mother's position. Some papers even comment that the cord floats. Yet the cord does not float; it sinks. The cord can find its way toward the cervix. It always falls away from the fetus even if the fetus chooses to handle it. This sinking property of the cord may be important in preventing cord entanglement. It may be nature's way of reducing the risk of the fetus harming itself. The cord usually bunches up in front of the fetus, commonly near its legs and feet. Long cords may make themselves more available to the fetus and enable the fetus to mouth the cord like a pacifier or handle the cord like a toy. Whether or not this is preferable depends on whether cord blockage is present during the sucking and handling. These simple fetal behaviors may play an important role in fetal well-being and development. Reflexes may exist that serve the purpose of short-duration cord play.

How hard a fetus can squeeze its fist at a given gestational age is unknown. Knowing whether the fetus can grab the umbilical cord and obstruct its own blood flow would be helpful. The grasp would have to exceed its own blood pressure and squeeze with a pressure greater than the fetal systolic pressure (60 mm Hg). Could the strength of some fetuses be a disadvantage? Could the thickness or thinness of cords predispose the cord blood flow to collapse if squeezed? Does the fetus faint and let go? Some anecdotal reports suggest that all these scenarios are possible. A long cord in and of itself is not dangerous. What becomes dangerous is the way in which the fetus interacts with its supply line. The Collaborative Project, a national study of over fifty-five thousand pregnancies, concluded that long cords are associated with fetal entanglement. The key here is to understand that entanglement depends on fetal repositioning in the uterus. Does the umbilical cord itself cause the problem, or does the fetus have to cause the problem? What does the fetus do to become entangled? Are there identifiable factors contributing to an active fetus (one which frequently repositions itself in the uterus and increases its chance of cord entanglement)? Lastly, what role does the mother play when she is active, and does diet play a role? Dietary factors and fetal behavior are currently being investigated. Maternal exercise is also being studied relative to its effect on the fetus. Fetal behavior over time is an active area of research. Scientists are looking for patterns that could mean the difference between well-being and illness.

> A better understanding of the physiology of pregnancy and labor has done away with the theories that the activity of the mother causes coiling of the cord. (Gardiner 1922)

Nuchal Cords: When a fetus's umbilical cord crosses itself 360 degrees around the neck, it has a nuchal cord. Dr. J. Selwyn Crawford of the British Medical Research Council first defined this problem in 1962 as the condition in which the umbilical cord is wound at least once around the neck of the fetus. This initial description was applied to a study that made the following conclusion:

> [The] nuchal cord is well recognized as being commonly associated with fetal distress and neonatal depression. It is all the more remarkable, therefore, that little work has been published to demonstrate the incidence of the condition, and to analyze its effects during labour and delivery. (Crawford 1962)

This finding was observed in 15% to 30% of nuchal-cord deliveries. Great variances of nuchal-cord observations exist because prenatal diagnosis with ultrasound has only recently been made. The accuracy of previous studies is in question because close adherence to specific definition may not have been followed. Nuchal cords are at the center of the supply-line controversy because so much differing information exists. To study nuchal cords, the fetus involved must be prenatally identified. Cords can wrap around the fetal neck as soon as the cord reaches four-fifths of the fetal length. This occurs as early as ten to twelve weeks' gestational age. Fetuses can entangle themselves multiple times; deliveries of fetuses with six to eight complete loops around the neck have been described. What distinguishes a surviving fetus from a stillborn fetus with a nuchal cord is unclear; however, some insights exist. For example, fetuses born dead with cords around the neck have been described from abortuses (eight to twelve weeks) to postterm (weeks). Yet no one clearly understands when these fetuses die, and no one has clearly observed those cord patterns. Actually, not all nuchal cords are the same. One researcher noticed a predisposition to nuchal-cord-related deaths around thirty-eight weeks. This is difficult

JASON H. COLLINS, MD, MSCR

to verify because ultrasound was not used to accurately date the fetuses. Another researcher noticed that two patterns exist: the cord crosses over itself, or the cord crosses under itself. This observation may be important when considering knot formations in the cord. A cross-under pattern is needed for knot formation and can cinch a nuchal cord if it rolls back on itself. Are multiple nuchal loops more deadly than single nuchal loops? Does the chance of fetal death increase with the amount of loops in the cord? Again, a definite answer is unknown, but many factors have been noted. Regardless of the number of loops, the problem lies in supply-line disruption. For example, fetuses who are breech are more likely to have more loops than fetuses who are vertex (head down). The shoulders of breech fetuses are freer to rotate than those who are vertex. Placental position is another factor. Activity, again, may influence the formation of nuchal loops. In addition, male infants seem more predisposed than female infants. There are also combinations of these factors. Nuchal cord formation is a function of fetal life. Once a cord is long, it is more likely to affect an active fetus. A very active fetus, especially one with a high level of amniotic fluid volume and a high level of energy derived from placental design, may be predisposed to nuchal cord formation. The number of infants killed by their umbilical cords is unknown. The National Center for Health Statistics does not have enough data to determine this. Possibly as few as four thousand deaths per year or as many as eight thousand deaths per year involve umbilical cord complications. The important point here is, these infants are normal; they are normal, but they are dead. Some researchers believe that cord accidents do not cause death. However, Dr. Arnold Lillien of NICHD explains this may not be correct.

> In general, however, the consensus of opinion has been that a nuchal cord is unlikely to compromise a fetus and is rarely, if ever, a cause of fetal death. We found a significant incidence of tight nuchal cords among term intrapartum fetal deaths without explanation. (Lillien 1970)

A similar opinion is shared by Torgrim Sørnes, MD, who has studied this issue for two decades. "The pathology of umbilical cord encirclements around the fetal body, neck, or extremities has not been subjected to thorough study for years, and little is known of their etiology, pathogenesis or effects on the fetus." (Sørnes 1995)

Cord Entanglement: The umbilical cord can surround an extremity, the body, or the neck. Body loops can be single or multiple and can exist with nuchal cords. The number of body-loop incidences is unknown. Most of these entanglements are undone at delivery as the infant is being born; therefore, they are never witnessed and never recorded. This lack of documentation in the medical record means, studies that use this information cannot be accurate. To date, PI's PUCP has this data.

The effect of a body loop is cord compression. Tight loops have made impressions on the skin of the fetus and can restrict fetal movement in the uterus. Loops around the extremity can affect circulation of the extremity and cause damage to a foot or a hand. Circulation disturbances can sometimes form blood clots in the arteries, vein, or placenta. These events can change the oxygen supply to the fetus and cause growth disturbances or death. Yet the variety and magnitude of cord entanglement become evident when one considers factors such as cord design, Wharton's jelly thickness, placental types, cord insertion sites, and fetal position. The explanation is not impossible and may be finite. There are no prenatally derived statistics that can provide the scope and incidence of cord entanglement. To arrive at this explanation, an understanding is needed of the number of prenatal incidences, the length of time that nonnuchal-cord entanglement lasts, and the effects on the fetus.

Combinations:

These experiments show that even a slack knot may be sufficient to interfere with, if not completely obstruct, the cord circulation, but that any pull upon the knot such as might be exerted if the cord were wound around the child's neck or body as to cause a relative shortening of it, would easily cause sufficient tightening to impede the circulation completely.

—Francis J. Browne, MD
Edinburgh Royal Maternity Hospital
Great Britain, 1923

Three cases of umbilical cord entanglement were described as complex (combinations). The cases were associated with intermittent fetal bradycardia, reduced fetal movements, and prematurely delivery.

Umbilical cord loops were around the neck, limbs, and body. Placental pathology showed downstream effects of cord occlusion and fetal thrombotic vasculopathy.

M Dodds, R Windim, J Kingdom
Ontario, Canada 2012

In addition to individual cord conditions creating fetal disturbances, potentially dangerous combinations are often observed. Yet the risk of harm is unknown. Whether a combined cord complication increases the chance of stillbirth compared to a single cord complication is unknown.

Another unknown is the effect the mother's toxemia or a disorder such as anemia may have on the fetus. Combinations involving fetal umbilical cord insertion-site hematomas (vessel rupture) have been observed. These hematomas were associated with nuchal loops, true knots, and midcord hematomas. These particular combinations suggest an umbilical cord subject to stretch mechanisms, possibly tearing the umbilical vein near its insertion. Reports of infants born with more than one knot and as many as three imply that fetal activity and repositioning are key factors. Were all three knots formed at once or one at a time? Is there a time during fetal development that is at highest risk for multiple knot formation?

The gestational age at which knots form would be valuable information so that increased screening could be initiated at that gestational age. Infants delivered with nuchal cords and a true knot are not uncommon. Upon closer inspection, the cord is usually long. The excessive length increases the probability of knot formation, but it is not necessarily deadly. Increased slack decreases the chance of tension. Cord architecture is also a factor. However, in studies that recorded length, cord type was not included.

Torsion: Torsion is the condition of the umbilical cord where twists are superimposed on the cord itself. Knots and nuchal cords are not always seen with torsion, but they can be observed with torsion. This combination, though, can be dangerous because cord positions that allow tension will cause torsioned cords to kink. Torsion is tolerable as long as the torque (imposed twist force) is released as a deformation of the cord (a snarl). If the energy of the snarl is reimposed, the cord blocks just like a garden hose. A deadly combination is a cord under torsion with a shoulder loop, nuchal cord, body loop, or extremity loop.

Finding vessel thrombus combined with torsion is not unusual. These thrombi can also be seen in the surface vessels of the placenta. Many of these combinations go unnoticed simply because no one is looking for them. When blockage occurs with cord-compression mechanisms, one of the clues left behind is edema (a buildup of fluid) of the cord. It is not unusual, for example, to have a nuchal cord with proximal cord edema, suggesting mild episodes of blood flow disturbance but not enough to cause death. In addition, it is not unusual for these combinations to cause fetal heart rate changes severe enough during labor to cause an emergency C-section. Short cords may be more dangerous because they are shorter, may marginally attach, and may be a velamentous insertion. This increases the chances of umbilical cord rupture compared to a normal insertion. Short cords may also predispose the cord vessels to thrombosis, hemorrhage, or hematoma formation. Individual reports of such occurrences are published in the medical literature. Although not common individually, all combinations as a whole present a significant occurrence when viewed on a larger scale. When combined, these events represent a more prevalent failure of reproductive mechanisms when compared to the most common genetic malformations. Altogether, in any community hospital practicing obstetrics, cord complications will be observed more often than congenital defects.

For instance, one medical review of just hematoma formation of the umbilical cord at Johns Hopkins Medical Center was observed in 1 out of 5,505 cases. Down Syndrome, a common genetic alteration known as trisomy 21 syndrome, occurs overall as 1 in every 660 deliveries. Trisomy 18, another readily acquired genetic defect, occurs as 1 in every 3,000 deliveries. Trisomy 13 occurs as 1 in every 5,000 deliveries.

Hematoma of the Umbilical Cord:

The causes of rupture of an umbilical vessel are obscure and probably several factors enter into the development of a hematoma in each case.
—A. Louis Dippel, MD

Johns Hopkins University and Hospital
Baltimore, Maryland, 1940

A hematoma of the umbilical cord is due to bleeding into the substance of the umbilical cord. They can be spontaneous, iatrogenically induced, traumatic self-induced, or secondary to an umbilical cord defect. The usual risk of cord hematomas that is often quoted is 1/1,000 to 1/5,500 rps deliveries. Hematomas can be due to the umbilical artery or umbilical vein. This sausage-shaped injury seems to be more frequently noticed on the fetal end than on the placental end. The chance of death to the fetus is as high as 50% and as low as 14%. The cause of hematoma development is unknown. Some scientific insights suggest wearing of the vessel walls, thinning of the walls, tearing, and then bleeding into the substance of the cord. Compression of the cord vessels leads to clogging and then death of the fetus. The sight of hematoma formation can vary, however. Again, unknowns exist in the area of umbilical cord hematomas. For example, it is unclear whether the cause of the fetal-end hematoma is the same as the placental-end hematoma. The most common time of hematoma formation is also unknown. Most discussions of formation have centered around labor and delivery. This would suggest that cord tension may play a role, and this tension can possibly be attributed to a condition where the cord is stretched. Obviously, observation of this condition was recognized long before recorded history and must have motivated many speculations. Since most modern reports (1871 to present) have described mostly stillborns, cord compression is an end result. Numerous descriptions focus on hematomas that originate from the umbilical skin. Vessels penetrating the Wharton's jelly from the umbilicus may rupture from fetal manipulation, which includes pulling on the umbilical insertion. Infants can grasp before birth and have been observed sucking and pulling on everything in the uterine amniotic cavity.

The most difficult feature of umbilical cord hematomas is that they are spontaneous and evolve quickly. Many case descriptions suggest that the fetuses were not in labor. More information is needed about the timing of these events and particular fetal behavior that may predispose the cord to hematomas if the fetus is vulnerable.

Torsion: As previously described, torsion is the condition of the umbilical cord where twists are superimposed on the cord itself, similar to an overly twisted telephone cord.

Umbilical cord torsion may not be an unusual finding. "In human beings, the umbilical cord is subject to many kinds of torsion, coiling, looping and knotting during pregnancy or during parturition. Torsion of the cord is a common occurrence." (Atwood 1932)

No formal definition of torsion currently exists. Veterinary scientific literature is quite familiar with the problem of torsion, especially in thoroughbreds. In fact, torsion is often a cause of fetal loss in horses. Veterinarians readily observe this finding and look for confirmation by studying other fetal structures confirming its presence as the cause of death. In one study of fetal losses in horses, 200/2,000 were due to this umbilical cord accident. Another topic more easily discussed in animal research is the association of torsion with heart failure and the finding of thromboses in the placenta. Clearly, torsion is readily accepted as a cause of fetal death in animals. For humans, this is not the perception. Some think that torsion occurs after death as a result of random movements of the dead fetus.

Prior to the Pregnancy Institute's study of torsion of the umbilical cord, no case report of a live birth with torsion existed in the medical literature. All descriptions of human umbilical cord-related torsion have been in stillborns. Therefore, the Pregnancy Institute's information did not come about easily. Dr. Kurt Benirschke, a Harvard-trained pathologist and professor emeritus of pathology at the University of California, San Diego, has provided us with invaluable insights into the mystery of this fetal/placental abnormality, especially torsion of the umbilical cord. He determined that the cord becomes intensely twisted, placental damage occurs secondary to thromboses, a common time of death is between twenty-eight and thirty weeks' gestational age, and torsion of the umbilical cord is seen in cerebral palsy cases. With this information, our observations of umbilical cord torsion began with normal live deliveries. Dr. Benirschke's suggestion of an intensely twisted umbilical cord prompted us to untwist the cord in over four hundred deliveries. We determined that torsion is actually very common but not always pathologic. Next, we determined the time in which pathology occurs and the spectrum of effects. The effect of torsion can be fetal harm ranging from heart failure to stillbirth. Torsion is not a natural state of the umbilical cord. Torsioned cords must not be confused with naturally helical, coiled, or spiraled cords. The appropriate terminology should be the word *helical*, which implies a constant, if not same, diameter. Torsion and natural helixes are different from each other. According to European literature, the curly course of the cord was considered in 1521, and left versus right (clockwise/counterclockwise) patterns were recognized in the 1600s. Left curls (80%) predominate over right curls (20%). Early estimates of total curls averaged eleven turns per cord (Hyrtl 1890). These estimates may be different from each other, however, because twists were not removed by unwinding. Most umbilical cords on the average (55 cm) have three to five helixes, the upper limit having eight helixes. The average number of twists is three. Together, the average curls could be Hyrtl's eleven. These same quantities are also found in equine cords. Cords can become twisted when the fetus repositions itself. Therefore, torsion is not an umbilical cord anomaly or abnormality. It is a mechanical deformation/alteration due to the behavior of the fetus. The importance of the formation of torsion implies much about intrauterine life and the dangers that face the fetus. These dangers are as significant as those that a newborn gazelle faces on the African savannah. The fetus begins to move around ten weeks' gestational age. If fetal activity is excessive, trouble begins. Torsion, nuchal-cord formation, body-loop formation, and true knots are related. The relationship depends on the type of repositioning that takes place. Fetuses can tumble, roll, and somersault like a gymnast in the three-dimensional environment. Torsion occurs when the fetus imparts these motions to the cord. This mechanical energy is called torque and is subject to the same laws of physics as any structure that is deformed by the same force. Twists occur as a result of this torque, and torsion occurs when twists involve every ninth a ratio of 1 twist per 5 cm or less of cord length. Torsion of the cord is a remarkable example of nature on the edge. For example, if a 50-cm cord has 10 twists imparted to it by thirty weeks, it can relieve the torque by growth of the cord. If the fetus remains in one position after thirty weeks, the cord could grow another 10 cm and change from a ratio of 1 twist to 5 cm (1/5) to 1 twist to 6 cm (1/6). The danger is therefore averted.

Collapse and kinking of the cord blood vessels seem to occur at a ratio below 1/5. The cord must then stretch so it can redistribute the stress/strain of the torque, which usually ends up being at a point near the placental end of the cord. A simple example is a telephone cord. Once heavily twisted, it narrows and snarls (loops over itself). Over time it becomes a complete mess. Torsion is an umbilical cord complication that is dependent on a number of factors. For example, fetal behavior is determined by intrauterine needs. This intrauterine fetal ballet has a purpose, function, and plan: get the fetus into a comfortable head-down prelabor position. The fetus may attempt this several times before reaching the milestone. Its success within a few attempts depends on placental position, amniotic fluid volume, inner ear (vestibular) maturation, and maternal diet and activity. If one of these factors is exaggerated, the fetus may begin the process of excessive activity, continued repositioning, and torque of the umbilical cord.

> Undue twisting of the cord (torsion not coiling), especially in that portion near the fetus where the Wharton's jelly is less abundant, probably can cause feta asphyxia. In the case illustrated, death of the fetus occurred about a week before delivery and was preceded by a period of *violent movements*. (Novak 1941)

Because torsion and its effects are also dependent on umbilical cord length, short cords may succumb faster than longer cords. Again, the type of cord may also play a role where type IV (vein around arteries) may be more prone to collapse under equal stress than other types (arteries around vein). Cord diameter/circumference also plays a role. A thicker cord may offer more resistance to torque than a thin cord. This is in need of study and will require a specialized vascular laboratory. Fetuses may also possess natural reflexes that allow them to untwist themselves. Cord helixes can be left and right in nature but mostly left (80%). If the fetus counterpositions itself, under favorable conditions of intrauterine life, it can get itself out of a perilous torsion. How often and in what way the fetus repositions itself during intrauterine life are unknown. One clue to this question is the twists seen at delivery. We have found that the average number of twists is $3\frac{1}{2}$. This was determined by untwisting over 300 umbilical cords at birth. It suggests that the fetus repositions itself in one direction 360 degrees ($3\frac{1}{2}$ revolutions). Unfortunately, the fetus may move in clockwise and counterclockwise directions. This would suggest that 6 moves left to right could be negated by 3 moves right to left, leaving the 3 twists as an inaccurate record. The fetus probably moves more often in the same direction and usually does not reposition itself often. Ideally, a constant

JASON H. COLLINS, MD, MSCR

series of ultrasound exams or a device that detects fetal position (like global positioning systems) might give us the final answer. Knowledge of the usual intrauterine activity over time would help solve the problem of torsion. [Insight—skin reference which would be trackable.]

Umbilical Cord Knots:

> The number of knots on the umbilical cord of a first born child is held to foretell how many of a family the mother is to have.
> —"Umbilical Cord Folklore"
> *The British Medical Journal*
> 1912

On first inspection, it is remarkable that a fetus can tie a knot in its umbilical cord. How is that possible? Monoamniotic twins (twins in the same sac) can create multiple knots together. No reports, however, exist that Siamese twins had knots in their common cord. This twin anomaly of reproduction suggests that the fetus must move to form a knot. Two separate fetuses moving independently create cord chaos, which can lead to multiple sites of constriction and fetal death. So how does a knot form, and what happens to the knot in utero? Most true knots are probably not formed before birth but during birth. It is highly likely that the fetus is entangled with the cord and, when delivered, is pulled through a loop of cord, forming a knot. To form a knot, the loop of cord must be special. It must be long enough for the fetus to form a nuchal cord. The nuchal cord must cross under itself, not over itself. This cross-under pattern allows the formation of a single hitch knot. The loop of crossed-under nuchal cord must pass over the fetal body before a knot can form. This specialized loop sometimes forms around an ankle and entraps it. The fetus is born with a snared ankle instead of a true knot. Sometimes both ankles can be involved. If the knot completes itself, the risk of blockage is great. We speculate that prenatal knots may form prior to thirty-two weeks, a common time of fetal repositioning. Yet the time at which most knots form prenatally is unknown. Knots may form earlier and have been noted prior to twenty weeks in miscarriage specimens. The earliest knot seen prenatally with ultrasound is in monoamniotic twins at nineteen weeks.

To envision knot formation, it is important to remember torsion. As the fetus repositions in the uterus, it applies torque to the umbilical cord; this energy causes the cord to loop counter to the direction of the torque, thereby crossing counter to the fetal movements. A cross-under loop has now formed, which, if lassoed around the fetal neck, can work its way along the fetal body to form a knot. The fetus may not even have to change position because its movements may work the loop to its feet and then off. Knot complexity depends on the amount of snarls created at the base of the loop. One snarl creates a single knot, two snarls a double knot, and three or more snarls a complex knot. Double snarls with double loops have also been described. The whole process is actually simple. A complex knot does not imply multiple fetal tumbles and twists. It only means the fetus passed through a loop or loops simultaneously. How the fetus can cinch a knot tight and block blood supply depends on other factors. As with a prolapsed cord, complete compression of blood flow will cause fetal harm. A knot can completely block the cord, and a knot can be tightened by the fetus during prenatal life. The chance of having a fetus deliver with a true knot of the umbilical cord is on the average 1% to 2%. The chance of fetal demise secondary to a knot blockage is 5% to 10%. It is not known whether the most common knot is a single, double, or triple knot. It is also unknown whether more complex knots are more deadly. It is known, however, that the chance of fetal death is increased with a knotted cord.

Body/Extremity Loops: Body and extremity loops, some of the more difficult mechanisms to observe, may be significant causes of fetal decompensation. Anecdotal reports have described extremities damaged by tight loops. The ability of these loops to injure an arm or leg but not cause fetal death is difficult to determine. Stillbirths are observed with multiple loops around ankles, necks, and bodies; yet it is difficult to determine which compressed segment caused death. Cord loops around the body are usually not observed because delivery unwraps them. The loop puzzle is pulled apart at the moment of delivery, so it goes unseen. The incidence seen at delivery is probably less than what actually takes place prenatally over time; probably 0.5% to 2% is reported. The increased chance of stillbirth is still debated. Chinese and Russian medical literatures tend to suggest that loops are not benign. If a fetus persists with a body loop, the chance of cord compression appears greater than if no loop exists. Body loops also can act like

JASON H. COLLINS, MD, MSCR

winches, taking up slack and causing relative shortness of the cord. This shortness may lead to placental separation and, in one report, maternal amniotic fluid embolism. Does a fetus recognize that its supply line is being compressed? Is there a fetal instinct that reacts to limitation of movement? Currently, some basic science experiments in rats suggest that this exists. Observations of entangled fetuses suggest the fetus is moving in one direction and not back and forth. Untangling a triple nuchal cord is usually in the same clockwise or counterclockwise direction in which it formed. Most loops originate over the fetal right shoulder and unwind counterclockwise. Similarly, torsion untwists clockwise. Fetuses may instinctively be preprogrammed to register favorable right-to-left rolls.

Whether this is totally reflex, chance, or instinctive evasive movements is unknown. The role of the inner ear (balance, orientation) vestibular system is also unknown. Could the fetus become faint or dizzy in utero? If so, does this cause unusual fetal movements that lead to tumbles/ somersaults and rolls? Can diet play a role? It is suggested that caffeine and xanthines (tobacco, chocolate, tea, coffee, soft drinks) may keep the fetus awake. Does this predispose the fetus to more activity and possibly more risk? Does the fetus develop a sense of position as well? After all, fetal hearing matures around twenty-four weeks. The fetus hears low-frequency sounds. The vestibular system is an ancient, evolutionary sense. Fish have had it for a long time. Is the fetus using its well-developed sense of position since its taste, smell, and sight senses cannot determine its orientation? If so, can its sense of position be disrupted by other stimuli and send it into a search pattern of disoriented movement resulting in body loops? How cord compression affects the fetus is discussed in the next chapter. How the fetus behaves and why it may be designed not to entangle itself will also be addressed next.

It is suggested that the reduced fetal movements and the changes in fetal heart rate were due to a diminished blood flow in the cord vessels as a result of gradual cord compression. (Sadovski 1976)

Three umbilical cord complications occur at least once in every four deliveries, and their problem cannot be avoided. (Spellacy 1966)

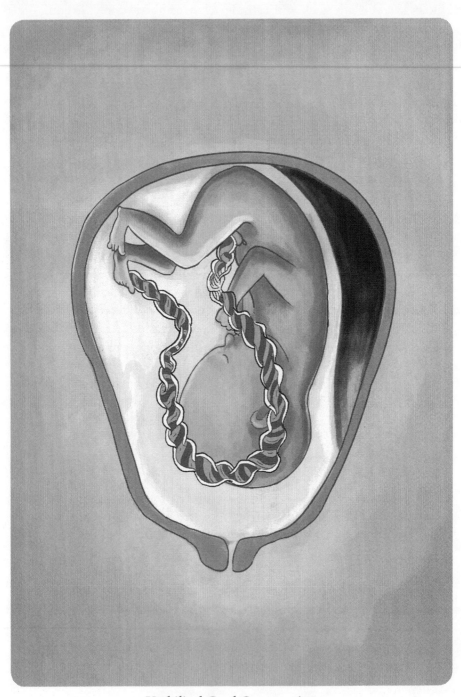

Umbilical Cord Compression

CHAPTER THREE

Fetal Behavior and Physiology

Whatever may be the final determination concerning the etiology of coiling of the cord, the movements of the foetus will undoubtedly play a prominent part in it.

—John Paterson Gardiner, MD
Toledo, Ohio,
1922

Any fetus that frequently changes position as found by routine examination is a candidate for torsion, looping, or knotting of the cord.

—James P. Hennessy, MD
New York, New York,
1964

Before the invention of ultrasound technology, much uncertainty surrounded the unseen developing fetus. How the fetus grows, moves, sleeps, and acts in the uterus was not certain. Ultrasonography allowed visualization of the fetus inside the mother as it transforms itself up to the moment of labor and delivery. Visually studying these behaviors has allowed for new insights. Fetal heart rate monitoring is the detection and recording of the fetus's beat-to-beat heart rate. This noninvasive electronic tool allows study of fetal reaction to its intrauterine environment under stressful conditions. Changes in the quality and character of the beat-to-beat pattern of the fetal heart allow graphic patterns to be recorded that translate into some basic fetal physiologic conditions. Fetal heart rate monitoring and ultrasound imaging together have contributed to the overall impression obstetricians have today of how the fetus works and interacts with the placenta, umbilical cord, uterus, and mother. Dr. Peter Nathanielsz, MD, PhD, has studied fetal development for the National Institutes of Health. He states, "Ultrasound shows us that each fetus has his or her own personality . . . . We can use ultrasound as a video camera on the developing fetus. We can track the fetus's heart beat and can follow his responses to sound and uterine contractures (uterine cramps which last 5 minutes) . . . . Ultrasound reveals the intricate systems which have evolved to allow human survival and continuation of life."

3-D and 4-D ultrasounds have the ability to view the fetus in more detail. More than thirty umbilical cord pathologies have been documented in peer-reviewed imaging literature. A new imaging tool, the MRI (magnetic resonance imaging), can also identify these pathologies. Ideally, the current eighteen—to twenty-week ultrasound study should include the fetus, placenta, and umbilical cord. It should state the placental position, site of cord attachment, type and length of umbilical cord (twisted versus straight), and fetal umbilical cord attachment.

To understand the fetal ballet of intrauterine life, a place to start is the shape of the uterus itself.

The uterus is neither globular nor cylindrical but bean-shaped. The bulge is created by the lower back (spine) as it bends forward (lordosis at 2 cm-4 cm) with pregnancy. Lordosis creates a central hump in the uterus that helps stabilize the fetus from excessive motion. It may serve as an obstacle to fetal rolling. Finally, this shape may guide the fetus to a head-down launch position by thirty-seven weeks.

Throughout pregnancy, this choreographed, instinctive behavior is directly linked to fetal survival. The fetus develops intrauterine reflexes to cope with maternal movements and positions. Without these abilities, the fetus will fail in its journey to birth. A new perspective on the fetus that is at odds with the old perspective has emerged in the last thirty years. The fetus is believed to be independent of the mother relative to its behavior. The fetus is also believed to control the onset of labor through its own local biochemistry, such as its endocrine and paracrine systems. These scientific facts put forth a view that the fetus is like a tadpole in a pond.

Amphibian eggs are laid and left to fend for themselves. The tadpole develops independent of the mother through multiple stages. The human fetus develops in the pond called the uterus without any direct maternal care. It must fend for itself. Thus, the fetus is an active participant in its development and environment, and it decides when it is born. It signals the mom to initiate labor, and part of that process is causing the release of melatonin from the maternal pineal gland from 9:00 p.m. to 6:00 a.m. This release is directly connected to uterine contractions, which is why most natural deliveries are at night. The fetus reaches milestones in the uterus just as a newborn reaches milestones of rolling, crawling, and walking over time. This scientific philosophy of fetal life points to behavior mechanisms of the fetus that would allow instinctive protection of the supply line (umbilical cord) by inherent reflexes. Evolutionary changes had to favor a combination of relative relationships that would allow success of a reproductive assembly such as ours. Mammalian species all have cord-related complications. Monkeys, horses, alpacas, and cattle have all been observed with umbilical cord problems. One difference is that these animals must be prepared to fend for themselves and ambulate at birth. The human is dependent at birth but is somewhat independent in the uterus. Cord compression can occur in the uterus. If labor begins (Braxton-Hicks contractions that can take three weeks), cord compression can intensify. The fetus can adapt to mild, infrequent cord compression and can resolve it. This can be observed using ultrasound, especially in pregnancies with multiple siblings, large uterine fibroids, and abnormal placental cord insertions, such as velamentous insertions and low-lying posterior insertions. This umbilical cord compression has associated reflexes and has been observed in animal models during controlled laboratory experiments. These experiments in pregnant rats and sheep fetuses that reproduce cord compression have observed fetal jerking movements, hiccups, and change of fetal position, which are believed to relieve the site of umbilical cord compression. These movements have been observed in human fetuses. It is believed that human single fetuses respond to cord compression with these reflexes. A type of human fetal-jerking movement has been described as a hiccup. These movements are rhythmical and last for ten to fifteen minutes. There should be two to three episodes in a twenty-four-hour period.

Dr. Joseph B. DeLee, professor of obstetrics, Northwestern University Medical School, wrote in his 1913 *Principles and Practice of Obstetrics* that hiccups were one of the most interesting phenomena of intrauterine life. The movements are short, quick jerks of the shoulders and trunk. In connection with these observations, he wrote that it was impossible to be sure that the infant was not suffering from asphyxia and was gasping for breath.

A later observer of this behavior was researcher John Patrick, MD (Toronto, Canada), who studied hiccups with ultrasound. He believed that three to four fifteen-minute hiccup episodes in twenty-four hours were normal. These episodes are observed beginning at twenty-six weeks and are diminished after thirty-two weeks. Hiccups are minimized toward term. A fetus having hiccups at term should be investigated. Do not assume frequent hiccups are OK.

A recent observation by Osamu Kurauchi, MD, of Nagoya, Japan, School of Medicine, supports the idea that startling, jumping, and writhing movements should diminish as the fetus matures. Studying anencephalic fetuses (without brains), he observed that as the fully formed brain matures, these activities are modified, and the behavior lessened toward term. In 1750, Dr. Smellie observed an infant with cord entanglement experiencing hiccups during vaginal delivery and afterward. We have reported that hiccups after three to four episodes lasting less than fifteen minutes in a twenty-four-hour period may not be physiologic and that more than three to four hiccup episodes occurring during maternal activity may suggest cord compression.

The nerve impulses that may cause hiccups may originate by way of the umbilical ring (belly button). Cholinergic and adrenergic nerve terminals, or end nests, have been identified in the umbilical cord 20 cm out and concentrated toward the umbilical ring. These nerve fibers run with the umbilical vein and sacral plexus to join the phrenic ganglion and celiac ganglion in proximity to the ductus venosus. The ductus venosus controls blood flow into the liver from the umbilical vein. It contains nerves and monitors fetal physiology. These fibers run with the vagal trunks and eventually may interact with the phrenic nerve by way of the medulla and respiratory center. The phrenic nerve sends fibers to the pericardium, phrenic ganglion, sympathetic plexus, and hepatic plexus. Compression or stretch of the umbilical cord may lead to spasm of the ductus venosus and contractions of the diaphragm similar to a reflex. This activity may be originating at the umbilical ring, which may be a pressure/blood flow sensor. These nerve pathways are basic structures of the human body and how it senses basic body functions. Fetal behavior is directly linked to its physiology and is based on reflexes (like an eye blink for dust irritation).

The way the fetus conserves oxygen, glucose, and water and its reaction to these altered elements are remarkable adaptations of an interactive life as compared to a more dependent development. The fetus is constantly faced with a changing physical compartment called the uterus. As the fetus grows and expands, it first encounters a cavity that is twice its size. Between implantation and twelve weeks, the fetus (embryo) remains on a short cord tether, thick and restrictive to motion; it also repositions and reacts to maternal activity. The fetus, therefore, is stable relative to its position. This is not the case after twelve weeks. As the uterus grows and the cavity becomes several times larger than the fetus by amniotic fluid expansion, the fetus now has "wings," extended arms and legs that are movable. Maternal activity can now distort fetal stability, and the fetus must respond to it or risk its supply line. Imagine an astronaut in space working on the space shuttle and spinning out of control. The line connecting life support to the shuttle will eventually fail. In intrauterine space, the fetus must develop a means to orient itself to react to maternal movements. This is accomplished by growth; fetal extremities resisting spin, roll, and tumble; and fetal reflexes adjusting fetal position. As the fetus matches uterine growth between twenty weeks and thirty-two weeks, fetal reflex responses and mass act like a disc brake to grab the intrauterine anatomy to stay put. The fetus can exercise and develop, but it is able to remain stationary and not reposition itself (similar to working a treadmill). There is a difference between fetal movements and fetal motion (repositioning). The fetus is designed not to roll, spin, or tumble because these motions are deadly. Fetal physiology as it applies to behavior of the fetus is primarily working to prepare the fetus for birth. It must have the ability to respond to changes that affect its heart rate, metabolic rate, neurologic status, and position. These alterations are the sources of fetal surveillance on which obstetricians depend to determine whether the fetus is compromised.

Fetal Senses

The main fetal senses are vision, hearing, touch, taste, and smell. Vision while developing is limited in utero. Eyelids are closed up until twenty-six weeks. Whether the fetus perceives light is unclear. At birth, newborns perceive shadows but do not clearly distinguish shapes. Vision would appear to be neither a primary mechanism for fetal behavior nor a means for the fetus to determine its position and status. In adults, vision is very important for day/night signals that manufacture melatonin and influence circadian rhythms. Fetal rhythms may be determined by maternal behavior and when meals are eaten.

Smell is not well developed at birth nor is taste, which depends on smell. Nose plugs exist during fetal life; therefore, smell would not determine how a fetus presents itself. Chemical markers are important to many animal species for identifying food, dangers, and each other. Yet for human fetuses, smell does not appear to play a major role in the uterus. Fetuses do not appear to identify parents by sight or smell at first. There is no need to forage for food in the uterus. Smell and taste only appear necessary in extrauterine life. Swallowing, however, is connected to intrauterine and extrauterine life. The fetus must swallow fluid to make urine and develop the gastrointestinal tract. Suggestions indicate that what the mother ingests may reach these fetal senses through the bloodstream. This backdoor chemosensory smell effect could play a role in how or whether the fetus ingests amniotic fluid.

What does amniotic fluid taste like to the fetus? Is the taste covered up by the chemosensory effects, like putting sauce on a steak? These answers are unknown; yet whatever the purpose, it is probable that these senses do not have the same role in intrauterine life. They may play a role in initiating labor by responding to meconium discharged to the amniotic fluid. Meconium is the product of the fetal intestines, which turns amniotic fluid green when expelled. Because meconium contains bile acids and other chemicals, ingestion may stimulate nerve receptors in the fetal nose and throat. These fetal nerve endings may contribute to neurologic signals reaching the hypothalamus, initiating the onset of labor. Touch is an important sense for the fetus. Our knowledge of fetal touch is understood by what we know about newborns. The rooting reflex appears to develop after birth. Before birth, this sense appears to work in the opposite way.

JASON H. COLLINS, MD, MSCR

For example, a fetus seen on ultrasound turns away when touched on the cheek. Sucking fingers, toes, and umbilical cords have also been observed on ultrasound. Yet turning away may be protective. Cord sucking may cause cord compression. In the uterus, turning away from objects may be beneficial. Touching and feeling the uterus, placenta, umbilical cord, and bony pelvis must be a part of fetal development. It may be a means for the fetus to locate comfort zones. Yet this may be more a function of pressure sensation than of feel sensation. It is believed that the fetus can feel at different degrees from head to toe. The head is more "sense mature" than the lower body and extremities. The fetus probably prefers to feel itself and spends a lot of time touching with its hands. Fetal grasping is reflex oriented. It is unknown how strong fetal grasp is (how much pressure it exerts). Can the fetus squeeze hard enough with its hand to occlude its umbilical cord with a pressure of 60 mm Hg or greater? It is also unknown whether touch or pressure influences fetal position. Hearing and position (vestibular) senses are related.

Another parallel sense is called kinesthetic sense or "Where are my body parts?" These neurologic developments are the results of millions of years of evolution. The oldest sense is vestibular (inner ear). Even before the appearance of man, fish have had a position sense. It is not known whether the fetus senses gravity, weight, and orientation. The nerves to the ear mature around twenty-four to twenty-six weeks. At this point, the fetus can hear low-frequency noises. It recognizes the maternal voice at birth. It may also have a sense of gravity (up/down). What role does hearing play in the uterus? Although the answer is unknown, we do know that the fetus can be startled with sounds in the uterus. These startle reflexes may play a role in controlling fetal position. Known startle reflexes, such as the Moro reflex, are usually described after birth. This pattern of fetal movement is well known and can be seen by shaking a newborn. The arms take on a hug position with the hands going out away from the body then inward.

What does this reflex look like inside the uterus? Imagine it as a fetal brake. The mother moves suddenly, and the fetus reaches outward to create contact between the uterus and itself. This has been observed on ultrasound, with the mother standing and lying. There are other startle-reflex patterns and fetal movements called tonic neck reflex, which extend the fetal arm, the opposite leg, and the head turns toward the extended arm. These reflexes are not intentional fetal movements as the fetus does not have coordinated movements. However, these movements do have an effect on helping the fetus change position. The vestibular mechanism may be connected to the startle reflexes to position the fetus and provide a means of avoiding cord entanglement. Neural systems connected to the kidneys and related to the midsection play a role in posturing independent of the spinal-cord input. These extravestibular gravity receptors may also be connected to the cardiovascular system through a major nerve called the vagus nerve. This connection is very important to fetal stability. Auditory senses may assist in neurologic development for birth and help provide parent recognition. How would these senses work to protect the fetus when it is active and asleep? When the fetus moves, it does so by movement of the midsection and the neck. These muscle groups are stronger than the extremities. It is often observed that the fetus kicks and jumps in utero. These activities are not coordinated and are not deliberately initiated by the fetus. When the fetus repositions itself as opposed to movements, different factors are involved. For example, the fetus may sense inner-ear pressure, which may change with position; the fetus may sense contours and prefer the left lateral position. In addition, auditory awareness of the placental souffle or maternal heartbeat may predispose the fetus to the head-down/left-lateral position. When uncomfortable, the fetus may attempt to roll, tumble, or somersault, using its startle reflexes to find comfort. This becomes more difficult after thirty-two weeks as the fetus is now larger than the uterine cavity and must fold itself into a fetal posture. If, in the process of repositioning, the baby becomes cord entangled, it may sense this through resistance to movement or the consequences of disturbed blood flow, oxygenation, and nutrient delivery.

Fetal Physiology as It Relates to Cord Compression

When the umbilical cord is compressed, the fetus immediately senses it. If the compression persists, the fetus will begin to undergo heart rate changes. These changes are sensed chemically (chemoreceptors) and physically (baroreceptors). The first response depends on how much of and how long the cord is compressed. Complete compression causes the fetus to notice changes in blood flow and blood pressure, oxygen decrease, and carbon dioxide accumulation. The heart slows, and the

JASON H. COLLINS, MD, MSCR

blood pressure rises. Eventually, this changes to a decreasing heart rate and decreasing blood pressure. Chemical signals are released to modify this response until it is corrected. Usually, a one-time, one-minute, 100% compression of the cord takes five minutes to completely correct. But within that one minute, oxygen levels have decreased 50%, and the fetus must reset the valuable energy and chemistry it has expended. In a recent experiment, complete cord compression for five minutes required thirty minutes for recovery. Continued five-minute compressions every thirty minutes caused fetal decompensation. This happens because the fetus cannot reset all its hormonal, chemical, and nutrient baselines quickly. Some refueling takes longer to rebuild than others. The main fuel of the fetus is glucose. The fetus has its own store of crystalline glucose called glycogen in the liver, heart muscle, and elsewhere, but it does not use this emergency supply unless it is completely deprived of maternal glucose. This is important for its survival and proper cardiac function if stressed. When the fetus senses blood flow interruption, it also senses a variety of organ reactions. The liver reacts by changing blood flow to a vessel called the ductus venosus. This vessel also directly connects the fetal heart to umbilical blood flow, providing the fetus with more oxygen than is already available. The fetus shifts blood from its extremities to favor enough oxygen to its heart and brain. If the blood flow derangement persists after one minute, other systems join in to adjust for the loss of oxygen and nutrients. In addition to liver blood-flow changes, the fetus experiences blood shifts away from its intestinal blood supply and kidney blood supply. Renal (kidney) blood flow is altered, which, if sustained, will begin to change renal function. Adrenal glands responsible for releasing stress hormones now secrete cortisol, a stress steroid, and immediate-acting adrenaline called catecholamines. These chemicals alter the fetus's cardiovascular system (heart rate, blood pressure, pulse) and stimulate the fetus to adjust its position if related to cord compression. This positional change would be invoked by the fetus bending its thorax and neck and by inducing hiccups. All the fetal reflexes are now initiated and modified to achieve normal state. Once these events take place, the fetus is probably tired, like an athlete running a sprint, and it needs to recuperate. As the fetus rests, its urine changes composition and becomes more diluted, releasing Na+K+Cl ions.

Similar events probably take place in the fetal intestine; however, if the fetus used liver and heart glycogen, it cannot be replaced. If the glycogen store is low, it could create difficulty for the fetus if it continues to be stressed and is unable to depend on its only fuel storage. Heart dysfunction could eventually take place.

Fetal Behavior and Physiology Secondary to Cord Compression

In animal models, usually fetal sheep, repeated complete blockage of the umbilical cord changes the way the kidney excretes basic electrolytes. These molecules are important for basic-cell-function K+Na+Cl ions. If the cells of the body are unbalanced, they do not work properly. Improper cell functioning is similar to having a bad stomach virus with diarrhea and vomiting. In addition, this change is connected to the secretion of a hormone called vasopressin. Vasopressin is responsible for moderating blood pressure. When the fetus is stressed, it attempts to change its function until it relieves the stress. If cord compression is not relieved, further physiologic changes begin—the purpose of which is to conserve oxygen. Blood flow can be taken from the extremities (arms and legs) and other organs (such as the lung) and preferably shunted to the brain and heart. This preserves the brain and heart at the expense of the body and gives the fetus time (ten to fifteen minutes) to solve the problem of obstructed umbilical blood flow. If the fetus cannot correct the cord blockage, final changes begin to unfold. The fetus can tolerate these conditions as long as it has oxygen and glucose and it is not losing blood. But beyond fifteen minutes, the fetus begins to decompensate and experience tissue damage. The most vulnerable tissue is nervous tissue. As the brain loses oxygen, it turns to a backup nutrient called lactic acid. The problem with this brain food is that it does not metabolize cleanly and leaves buildup molecules called carbon dioxide; this situation causes the brain to swell, prompting blood vessels to close. Brain damage then occurs. The degree of damage depends on many factors, such as the age of the fetus at the time and the degree of oxygen loss to the tissues. As the lack of oxygen increases, the heart begins to fail. Not only does it malfunction in its role as a pump, but it also begins to short-circuit and develop arrhythmia, which is irregular heartbeats. These electrical-conduction defects put the fetus at risk for heart stoppage. If the fetus is low on oxygen (hypoxic), high on lactic acid and carbon dioxide (acidotic), and experiences heart arrhythmias, it will die. The fetus has behavioral patterns that can create cord compression and release. These reflex movements and organ adaptations have evolved over millions of years.

The overall relationship is a vigorous fetus having the ability to develop in the uterus without injuring itself, its cord, or its placenta while growing. The process of labor alters all these behaviors and recruits a new set of protective mechanisms designed to evade disruption of the supply line. During labor, compression patterns can change from a single short episode to repetitive cord compressions to prolonged compression where complete blockage forces immediate delivery. A typical example of complete blockage is a prolapsed cord where the cord enters the vagina before the fetal head. The cord can be compressed between the bony fetal head and bony maternal pelvis. Usually, fetal compromise will occur if delivery does not take place in ten minutes. A more detrimental accident is blood loss. Placental separation due to a short cord, umbilical cord rupture due to a defective cord, or a ruptured umbilical vein hematoma prompts not only blood loss but a lack of oxygen as well. These types of accidents can cause fetal death in minutes. Little can be done under these circumstances as these infants need immediate, rapid treatment with blood, fluids, oxygen, and support. If they survive, it is usually with damage. The animal model, which is not familiar to most, is the one that simulates intrauterine, prelabor, intermittent partial cord compression. This will be discussed in the next chapter.

> Management and treatment options for umbilical cord complications will follow an understanding of the basic pathophysiologic mechanisms. (Mann 1986)

> We rely greatly on information from animals; too much since there are great variations between species we know so little; measurements of flow of the umbilical (cord) are imprecise, and we have few measurements of human fetal arterial blood pressure, or of its changes with age . . . . Hence, much is speculative! (Dawes 1995)

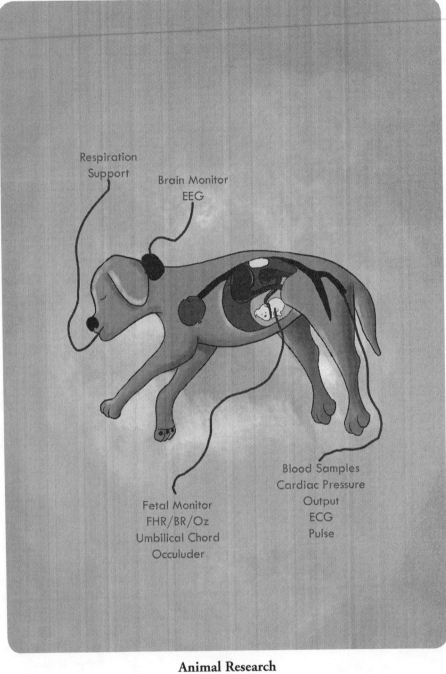

Respiration
Support

Brain Monitor
EEG

Fetal Monitor
FHR/BR/Oz
Umbilical Chord
Occuluder

Blood Samples
Cardiac Pressure
Output
ECG
Pulse

Animal Research

CHAPTER FOUR

What Animal Research Teaches Us about Umbilical Cord Accidents

Animals will continue to be as vital as the scientists who study them in the battle to eliminate pain, suffering, and disease from our lives.
—Heloisa Sabin speaking about
Albert B. Sabin and polio vaccine research
"Animal Research Saves Human Lives"
Wall Street Journal, October 1995

Some of our knowledge about how the fetus behaves and is affected by supply-line disturbances comes from animal research. The ability to solve the problem of umbilical cord accidents may depend on future efforts involving research in animal models. From mice to rats to dogs to sheep to primates, valuable insights may only be possible using these heroes of research. Numerous dedicated world-class researchers depend upon animal models for their work. Many have contributed invaluable insights into how the fetus works. Translating animal-model research results to humans is not perfect and, at times, very different. Sometimes, too, human research gives insights to help animals. An important animal model for fetal physiologic research is the fetal sheep. This works out fairly well due to sheep tolerance of manipulation and similarity of human biology. Through sheep, scientists study fetal reaction to various forms of oxygen deprivation—one of the more poorly understood areas of obstetrics. Fetal sheep can be chronically oxygen depleted or acutely oxygen deprived, and the response to each situation differs. The time in gestational weeks and duration of a lack of oxygen in these models can be varied to show different fetal responses. There are several ways to study these events. One is to limit oxygen to the mother of the fetal sheep while the mother is under anesthesia. This, in turn, limits oxygen to the fetus. Another method is to limit blood flow to the uterus. Special techniques exist to reduce placental blood flow and simulate intrauterine growth retardation, which is thought to be due to similar conditions. Direct blockage of the umbilical cord can limit blood flow and oxygen delivery in varying degrees. These studies help scientists understand all the ways a fetus can be compromised. A specific animal model in sheep fetuses blocks the umbilical cord to simulate umbilical cord accidents. Several such studies have suggested insights into how supply-line interruption affects the heart, brain, kidneys, and metabolism of fetal sheep. When the umbilical cord is compressed in these models, characteristic fetal heart rate changes take place. One pattern type is called variable decelerations. Variable fetal heart rate decelerations are changes in heart beat-to-beat patterns that cause the heart rate to decline below normal levels (110 beats per minute). This is also a clinical sign used to determine whether a fetus needs immediate delivery. To understand how this works, fetal lambs had occluders placed around their umbilical cords while in the uterus. The occluders were opened and closed by timed pumps to simulate possible intrauterine events. Highly specialized, sophisticated equipment were used to measure the oxygen, acidity (pH), and other chemistries of fetal physiology. These studies showed fetal stress within the first thirty minutes of a two-hour experiment. The fetal heart rate reacted immediately, and the body chemistry changed quickly. Characteristic heart rate patterns called W signs, U signs, and V spike signs appeared. Fetal stress hormones began to rise and eventually became depressed or modified. In the sheep fetus, this suggests that time is an important factor when umbilical cord compression is occurring. Considering this on a human level, correction of cord compression over a reasonable amount of time is important. If the human fetal heart works like the sheep fetal heart, then neurological regulation of the fetus deteriorates with progressing acidemia and hypoxia caused by these compressions. Even if fetal death does not occur, the effects on the heart may be enough to permanently change the heart muscle. For example, a drop in fetal blood pressure creates a decrease in coronary blood flow and O2 delivery directly to the muscle. Indirectly, chemical products from the placenta abruptly enter the heart after release of cord compression. These, in turn, can affect the heart muscle with modified oxygen called oxygen free radicals. This excited molecule can burn heart muscle and change it. Vitamins such as C and E are called free radical quenchers. They can react with the excited oxygen molecule and return it to a normal state.

The chronically instrumented pregnant sheep and fetus have been used to study the effects of umbilical cord compression on neurologic function (figure 40). An overall view of complete cord compression showed an increasing tendency of the fetus to conserve blood flow between the heart and the brain, using oxygen from the limbs. This, in turn, directs oxygen to the more fragile neurologic tissue and away from the more durable gastrointestinal tract, muscle, and skeleton. This diversion appears to protect the brain and heart in that it buys time for a correction (see chapter Three).

These experiments give scientists a chance to look at the brain's reaction to cord compression. For example, depending on time, duration, and degree of blood flow interruption, various changes are seen. One change is edema (swelling) of the brain tissue. If severe, edema can be damaging. It is known that normal infants with uncomplicated births have edema for several days. How all this affects the fetus at different ages is unknown since animal models in mature sheep suggest that umbilical cord compression can cause varying types of damage with different insults of oxygen deprivation. Complete cord compression with complete loss of blood flow and oxygen may have several effects in term infants. In term sheep, these events cause hippocampal (learning center) damage after 10 to 15 minutes. Striatal (neuronal) damage occurs after repeated 5-minute compressions. This area contains white matter and is located lateral to the ventricles of the inner brain. Important cross connections to the brain's right and left hemispheres are located in the striatum. In different experiments, 50% blood flow interruption caused brain swelling, heart rate changes, and endocrine changes. Brain edema can press small blood vessels on the underside of the brain against the ridges of the skull and selectively reduce blood flow to specific areas. Heart rate changes can lead to arrhythmia of the heart and heart stoppage. When the cord is clamped and released over time in term sheep, other patterns of damage occur in the (white) brain matter. Similar patterns have also been observed in primates. In addition to neurologic changes, blood flow shifts from fetal organs and extremities to the placenta and heart are also documented (figure 41). These patterns are important to define if the mysteries of cerebral palsy and learning deficits are to be understood. During the 36th to 40th week of human gestation, significant damage appears to be possible due to combinations of hypotension, hypoxia, and stress caused by prolonged cord compression. While the fetal heart and brain are being protected during cord compression, the fetal adrenal gland is also being protected. The adrenal gland sits atop the kidney and provides stress hormones and chemicals. The adrenal gland usually reacts to danger in a fight-or-flight manner. For example, if stressed or compromised, the adrenal gland can turn on the launch signal prior to its due date. In the sheep fetus, when cord compression reduces blood flow, extremity (limb) circulation is shunted in part to the adrenal gland. This enhanced blood flow allows chemicals from the gland to be excreted to the fetus. The gland has two parts: an inside core and an outside capsule. The immediate response is to produce adrenaline (norepinephrine, epinephrine). These chemicals raise fetal blood pressure and stimulate the fetal heart to beat faster. In fetal rats, it may cause the fetus to jerk or move. While this occurs, the adrenal gland produces a stress hormone called cortisol, which protects the fetus from collapsing or having a nervous breakdown. These chemical signals go to the brain of the fetus that, in turn, sends signals to the mother that may ultimately cause release of oxytocin and, perhaps, vasopressin, all of which may initiate contractions.

The liver is another organ that may be stimulated during umbilical cord compression. An important fuel for fetal life that is stored in the liver is glucose. This is in crystalline form and presents in muscle and other tissues. One study examined glucose metabolism in fetal sheep and noticed increased glucose hormones (glucagon and insulin) during decreased O2 exposure. The placenta, cord, and muscle contain glycogen that, once used, is not restored. In chick and mouse fetal heart samples, the distribution of glycogen inside the cell changes with time. With maturity, glycogen increases in the cell structure called the mitochondria. This is the cell engine and provides energy for cell mechanisms. Muscle-cell glycogen stays about the same over time. The overall glycogen in the cell decreases from one day to thirty as if concentrated in the mitochondria. Only when the fetus turns to a postdelivery metabolism can it rebuild glycogen. This change in stored fuel may be important for other fetal conditions.

JASON H. COLLINS, MD, MSCR

In addition, vessels in the liver tend to direct blood flow through an important vessel in one of several fetal shunts that are not needed after birth. Blood flow shunts are special vessels that redirect blood flow during fetal life. (Once born, these vessel detours are permanently closed to allow adult life.) Disturbances in these shunts may play a role in sending signals to the adrenal gland during stress through the right phrenic nerve. This nerve branch, which matures by twenty-four weeks' gestational age, could be an important emergency alarm that plays a role in quickly turning on stress chemicals when necessary. Umbilical cord compression also has direct effects on these shunts and their ability to stream blood to the heart.

Lungs are affected by these changes of blood flow through shunts in sheep animal models. Cord compression of 50% reduces lung interstitial blood flow. By altering O2 delivery, different patterns of damage are established. One of the effects of cord compression on lungs is the associate development of persistent pulmonary hypertension. This pathology has been demonstrated in a sheep model. A recent computer simulation model found that as the fetus shunts blood from the lower body to protect the brain and heart, lung oxygenation falls acutely. All current published facts point to a relationship between altered umbilical blood flow and lung maldevelopment.

Other lung effects unaddressed are fluid balance and surfactant production. The lungs are bathed in amniotic fluid, which participates in lung alveolar (air sacs) growth. It is unknown whether disturbances in water management can change the lungs' ability to mature. If the forty different lungs' cells are not receiving proper blood flow, they may not be producing chemistry to support lung functions such as O2/CO2 exchange. If fluid management is disturbed too much or there is too little fluid may alter how the fetus will breathe at birth. To date, no studies exist that consider amniotic fluid/lung function and relationships with chronic cord compression.

Thanks to expert studies of animal models, fetal responses to umbilical cord compression are known. A basic understanding of vital organs such as the brain, heart, kidney, lung, and adrenal gland will help determine how to help the stressed human fetus. The ability to study blood samples from both the mother and fetus will lead to methods to test the fetus and find the one needing delivery.

Some of the biochemical changes that can result from umbilical cord stimulation are as significant as organ, blood flow, and neurological changes. As the fetus experiences more stress, the tissues of the umbilical cord can secrete chemistry to react to the changes taking place. The local tissue reactions may be premature changes that would occur only during labor. Because the tissues cannot individually tell the difference, many false starts can take place. Local reactions in the umbilical cord by molecules released from the cells that line the umbilical vessels can cause momentary constriction or closure of the vessels. At birth, these molecules permanently close those vessels to prevent blood loss.

These small dynamic systems are constantly in balance. Thousands of these systems probably exist—some more immediate and more important than others. These systems are sometimes called autocrine and paracrine modulators, and they regulate local (cellular) chemical reactions. An obstetrical interest is the potential for a remedy to maintain blood flow. Discovery of a modulator that can be infused to the mother would be beneficial when there is evidence of blood vessel constriction. Animal-tissue studies can greatly enhance the understanding of these molecular effects. Studies in both human-tissue cultures and animal-tissue cultures have broadened our knowledge of umbilical cord-vessel endothelial cells. These are cells that coat the inside of umbilical arteries and veins. They produce the chemicals that respond to the conditions that occur moment to moment with the events of the placenta and fetal physiology.

LIST OF SOME PARACRINE/ENDOCRINE/AUTOCRINE MOLECULES

Oxygen—Several forms (modulators of other molecules)

Nitric Oxide—Relaxes placental vessels

Nitrite—Byproduct of oxygen and nitric oxide—inactive

Peroxynitrite—Byproduct of active oxygen—toxic to cells and active in the membrane of cells

Prostacyclin—Vasodilates placental vessels

Thromboxane—Constricts placental vessels and modulates coagulation

Endothelin-1—Constricts placental vessels

Epidermal Growth Factor—Tissue modulator

Poostanoids—Modulate coagulation of blood in umbilical vessels

JASON H. COLLINS, MD, MSCR

Prostaglandins (PGE2)—Constrict umbilical vessels at birth
EGF + TGF—Constrict and regulate cord function
Xanthine/Purines/
Adenosine—Vasodilates placental vessels
Catecholamines—Stress molecules that modulate vessels
Nicotine—Vasoconstrictive
Caffeine—Unknown
Chocolate—Unknown
Herbal Tea—Unknown
Anesthetics-Bupivacaine—constriction of umbilical vessels
2-chloroprecaine—dilation of umbilical vessels

It is known that the amounts of these autacoids differ from umbilical vein to umbilical artery and from the placenta to the fetus. Anticoagulation autacoids (blood thinners) are higher in the umbilical vein; vasoconstrictor autacoids are concentrated toward the fetus, which means that they are important in stopping blood loss from the cord when it is severed. Epidermal growth factor, which makes PGE2, is located less on the placental end than the fetal end. This difference allows the constriction of cord vessels to begin at the placental end and peristalsis (squeeze) of blood toward the fetus. This trick of nature ensures an adequate blood count for the fetus. If this fails in large animals such as cows and horses, the newborn calf or foal will die of shock due to lack of blood volume.

Numerous regulators also exist outside and inside the umbilical cord. Amniotic fluid contains molecules from fetal metabolism, and blood circulating through the cord has molecules that are important to blood flow. It is amazing that any of us are born in one piece. These multiple systems can remain in balance and can adapt to disturbances. What is unknown is the limit of that adaptation. When does failure begin, and how long after failure does damage begin? Sometimes damage is immediate, sometimes it is confined, and sometimes it is chronic. To know these answers is to discover important ways to protect the fetus at risk. Animal models also allow research into other reproductive byproducts such as the placenta.

Determining the effects of fetal derangement on placental function is most important. Where the fetus can avoid injury, the placenta may not.

No matter how vigorous the fetus is, it is in danger when the placenta deteriorates. The differences in placental structure from animal to animal allow varying effects. Sheep have multiple placentids where monkeys have one placenta like humans. Chimpanzees are better examples of human placental design.

Morbidity
Other Effects

Placental changes are important to study separate from fetal effects. These placental changes may or may not add to the fetus's ability to tolerate intermittent umbilical cord compression. The placenta has large reserves similar to other organs, where loss of placental tissue may be comparable to a loss of hearing in one ear, sight in one eye, or function of a kidney. The fetus can function and survive, but it may not grow and develop to 100% of its capacity. Cord compression may be a stimulus to induce such a compromise. It is theorized that if the umbilical blood flow is slowed, then placental blood flow is also slowed. When this happens, blood thickens in the small spaces in the placenta called the villous vessels and clots like gelatin. This, in turn, causes thromboses of the intervillous space that contains blood flow from the mother. The result is devitalized placental tissue and loss of that placental nutritional space. If enough dead space is developed, the fetus can be compromised. Thus, an indirect effect of cord pathology may be the secondary injury of the placenta even if the fetus does not, itself, become primarily injured. The umbilical cord complication observed that causes such a pattern is torsion (figures 42 and 43).

Animal placentas have been studied where torsion caused stillbirth of thoroughbreds (figure 44). Thrombi were seen in these placentas along with thrombosed surface vessels. Human placentas have been observed in cases of torsion where surface vessels were similarly thrombosed. The finding suggests multiple small blood-flow derangement episodes prior to death. Does this mean these events can be prenatally detected? It is possible that one day, ultrasound or maternal blood sampling will detect these changes. Another placental change that is more extensive than infarction of tissue is called chorangiosis. It is suggested that this change is due to low oxygen levels in the fetal circulation. This alteration of

JASON H. COLLINS, MD, MSCR

placental blood vessels looks like a rash. The vessels are dilated and full of blood cells. This change allows more surface area to grab more oxygen from the mother.

How much change is tolerated before fetal harm occurs is not clear. Chorangiosis and similar placenta changes have been studied in llamas and goats from high altitudes, especially in Chile. Because of low oxygen tensions at elevations above ten thousand feet, these animals provide an important insight into adaptations to tolerate chronic low-oxygen states. These changes seem to suggest that the chronically hypoxic (low oxygen level) fetus compensates with blood flow and blood cell expansion. To see similar changes in a fetus with cord entanglement suggests similar principles are involved.

All in all, multiple questions must be answered to solve the mysteries of umbilical cord compression. The answers may be forthcoming in each method of animal modeling used. Because of each unique characteristic of each species, study of the whole assemblage will be necessary to define umbilical cord-compression effects on the fetus.

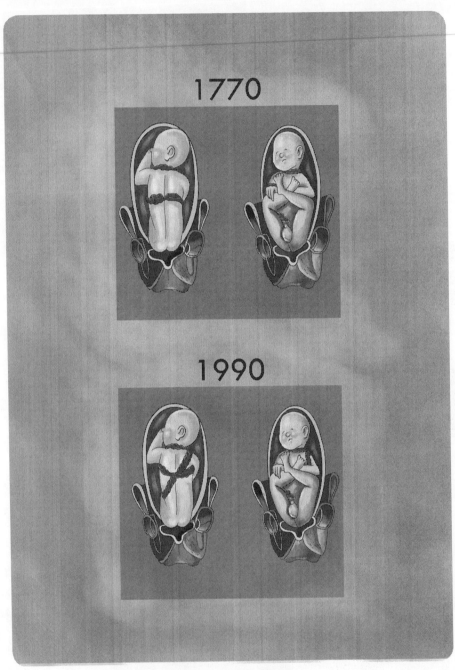

Umbilical Cord Entanglement

CHAPTER FIVE

Management of Umbilical Cord Anomalies, Abnormalities, and Complications

Fetal loss from umbilical cord abnormalities a difficult case for prevention.

—A. Ghosh, MD
Queen Mary Hospital
Hong Kong, 1984

"The baby who cheated death by 30 minutes: Doctors spot umbilical cord strangling foetus during routine scan and carry our emergency C-Section at 32 weeks."

Lucy LA,
Mail Online, May 12, 2013.

Managing the umbilical cord during pregnancy, labor, and delivery needs more discussion in obstetrical forums. In 1989, a publication from the US Department of Health and Human Services entitled *Caring for Our Future in the Content of Prenatal Care* describes specific pregnancy conditions or hazards. It comments that "structural abnormalities of the placenta are significant causes of poor pregnancy outcome." No other specific mention of umbilical cord-related events is listed, and no specific screening or management is suggested. This report of the Public Health Services Expert Panel on the Content of Prenatal Care did not address the issue of umbilical cord accidents but seemed to acknowledge an association with fetal harm. Increased discussions of cord-accident management are also important because this topic is virtually undeveloped and poorly defined. This fact is concerning because more infants are affected with cord complication than are with polio, AIDS, SIDS, pregnancy hypertension, gestational diabetes, or B-strep. The effects of umbilical cord-related complications can be as dramatic as a term stillbirth or as subtle as learning disabilities. It is consistent in that fetuses are being lost to cord accidents on a daily basis. The problem must not be understated. Once it was discovered that the polio virus caused harm, Dr. Salk was able to construct a management solution called polio vaccine. Umbilical cord accidents are causing stillbirth, asphyxia, emergency C-sections, fetal distress, and neurologic damage, which may consist of learning disabilities and cerebral palsy. How are these fetal harms to be prevented? Part of the difficulty in prevention seems to be in believing that an association exists. These relationships are difficult to demonstrate statistically. One analysis of cerebral palsy infants stated that looking at cord prolapse, body loops, and long cords, there were significant associations. All these insights are difficult to prove because the reviewed and relied-upon information is incomplete and full of statistical pitfalls. What can be done at this moment in time is to discuss and make clear the potentials of umbilical cord accidents. The attempt to manage cord problems during labor may go back to Zi-Ming Chen (AD 1237). His suggestion was to remove a shoulder loop by hand. "Doctor should ask the mother [to] lie on her back and be at rest, gently press its shoulder downward, and strip off the cord. Don't order the mother to exert her strength till the fetus positions itself properly."

In 1741, British obstetrician Dr. John Burton described several cases of cord management where delivery was impeded by a short cord and' an entangled cord. "I was sent to a patient at Healey Manor who had been in labor about 30 hours . . . . I did imagine that the umbilical cord must be too short, and then I reached the string and found it fully stretched with the placenta strongly adhering to the womb. I therefore broke the string [cord] and delivered the woman . . . . I was sent to a person at Enwood . . . . I introduced my finger a little further and found the umbilical cord sat about the child's neck. I therefore twisted that part of the cord, which reached from the child's neck to the placenta, about my two forefingers and with my thumb broke it, withdrew my hand, when the child soon followed."

Dr. Nelson Sackett in 1933 described a case where he reached inside the uterus, encountered two loops around the baby's neck, and extracted the infant in the back position (version extraction), rupturing the cord in the process.

A study reviewing over one thousand births recently concluded: "From the point of avoidability of prenatal deaths, this study indicates that there is no clinical pattern and therefore no place of treatment for the obstetrician to save those babies which are killed by their own umbilical cord." (McLellan 1988)

This conclusion was based on traditional obstetrical care. There was no attempt to use tools such as ultrasound and fetal monitoring as a preventative measure. Some researchers have taken a different approach. In a case report of a stillborn with a nuchal cord × 2 and true knot, Dr. M. Maneschi (Universitad di Palermo, Sicily) in 1977 recommended that "a situation of this kind could be suspected on the basis of certain clinical findings to be elicited by questioning the patient about the intensity of active fetal movements, as well as in the presence of changes of position of the fetus and the findings of a high presenting part at term. If on the basis of these findings the cord is suspected to be short, either in itself or as a result of coils around the fetal neck or body and if low placental insertion and other causes of the high position of the presented part have been excluded by echography (ultrasound) further tests can be carried out."

Recently, Dr. N. V. Strizkova, chair of the Department of Obstetrics and Gynecology, Moscow Institute, and Dr. S. M. Petrikovsky, obstetrical professor, University of New York, used endoscopic devices in 1981 to visualize fetuses in the uterus with cord entanglement during labor. Their solution was helpful in determining fetal risk once the membranes were ruptured. This attempt to manage the umbilical cord was followed by several scientific reports from China, Europe, Japan, and the United States, demonstrating ultrasound could visualize the umbilical cord.

Specifically, in 1982, P. Jouppila, MD (Oulu, Finland), described the ability to visualize the umbilical cord around the fetal neck. "Antepartum diagnosis of cord coilings would be of clinical value for the adequate suppression and management of this complication," he wrote. As ultrasound technology improved, more and more anecdotal reports appeared. Today it is recognized that ultrasound can visualize cord entanglement, abnormalities, hematomas, varices, knots, and architecture.

In a 1989 review by Dr. Ingo Clausen, professor of obstetrics and gynecology, University of Aarhus, Denmark, structural anomalies of the umbilical cord were mentioned as being diagnosed with ultrasound. Worldwide recognition that these potentially dangerous mechanical and acquired cord complications are responsible for antenatal fetal deaths is encouraging in that a solution and means of management are possible. Ultrasound visualization of cord position, structure, and function can be displayed in several forms. Black-and-white (grayscale) ultrasound can identify the outline (edges) of the cord and reveal the arteries and vein. Comparison to the fetus and placenta can detail both attachments and position. Doppler color ultrasound can visualize blood flow in color and outline the cord in red, blue, and yellow colors, depending on the direction of the blood flow. The two techniques provide a clear picture of cord condition relative to the fetus. The first step in managing the umbilical cord is visualizing it, and it can be visualized as soon as it forms. Measurements of the umbilical cord can begin as early as six to eight weeks. Knowing the length of the umbilical cord over time can help diagnose short or long cords and thereby anticipate difficulty with labor. Umbilical and placental insertion sites and characteristics can be visualized with ultrasonography. In addition, it is possible to visualize an abnormal placental insertion or an umbilical cord defect. The diagnoses of these cords have been described in many writings to date. Knowing that an abnormal insertion site exists may direct the obstetrician to look for growth disturbances.

In 1995, Dr. Torgrim Sørnes (Akershus Central Hospital, Norway) suggested that "there is an association between cord encirclement and fetal weight deviations, independent of cord length (effects)." An intense follow-up should be done on these fetuses. Another observation of cord abnormalities and fetal effects by Dr. John Rolschau (Odense, Denmark, 1978) states, "It has been documented that a thin umbilical cord is associated with low birth weight . . . Also, the RNA/DNA ratio was increased, indicating tissue stress (in the placenta) in cases of battledore insertions of the cord." Few studies have observed large numbers of infants from conception to delivery with these findings. This is necessary if the effects are to be accurately determined. A means of determining prenatally entangled fetuses having difficulty is needed. Case reports have been

JASON H. COLLINS, MD, MSCR

published on an individual basis where fetuses were prenatally observed with ultrasound and delivered when believed compromised. Torsion can be recognized by measuring the distance between the veins (pitch). A close pitch suggests multiple twists and the need to pay close attention to the fetus. Knowing which fetuses have the potential for umbilical cord complications is the next most important means of management is counting fetal movements. The mother can play an important role in preventing a tragic loss from a cord accident. While it is unknown how much time is needed for a fetus to die, it is believed that in most instances, the fetus dies slowly. As described earlier, fetal behavior is consistent, and if recognized by the mother, changes in fetal movement patterns can be documented and reported to the physician. Dr. E. Sadovsky studied movement among fetuses with cord complications and felt there was a pattern to signs of fetal stress. Older literature describes decreasing activity of the fetus over time. It is important for the mother to recognize when the fetus plays and when it sleeps. These activities should remain similar from thirty-two weeks until forty weeks. In addition, fetal strength should remain similar. However, fetal movement decreasing over time and weaker movement over time suggest fetal stress and should alert the mother to see her physician. Fetal jerking movement over time should also alert the mother. In addition, daily hiccup behavior (more than four episodes in twenty-four hours) suggests cord compression and initiation of fetal reflexes. These signs of probable fetal entanglement and/or placental insertion/location abnormalities should motivate the physician and mother to begin a surveillance plan, especially prior to forty weeks. All detections of changes in fetal behavior noted by the mother or the physician should be shared with each other.

The second step is to measure (quantitate) fetal behavioral change. The simplest way is to evaluate the fetal heart rate, or FHR. FHR recordings of fifteen-minute strips can be invaluable during prenatal visits. Comparison over time can help identify a stressed fetus. The most sensitive indicator of fetal physiology is the heart rate pattern and characteristics. Fetal heart rate patterns change immediately with cord compression. Degree and duration of cord compression are unique. These patterns (called lambda signs, V shape, W shape, U shape, variable decelerations, late decelerations, and overshoot) indicate fetal blood flow disruption. Patterns that repeat themselves and develop frequently suggest a compromised fetus. These pregnancies can be identified and studied. One method is to evaluate the FHR at home at least once a week with a fetal monitor. This may allow the discovery of a slowly deteriorating pattern that indicates delivery. Potential delivery is suggested with the detection of a double nuchal cord, an abnormal FHR pattern at thirty-eight weeks, and a change in movement patterns for twenty-four hours.

It is well known that by thirty-six to thirty-eight weeks, the fetal colon is capable of peristalsis (movement) and contains bile acids for digestion, debris from swallowing vernix/lanugo, and cells. This intestinal mixture is called meconium. It is believed that the fetus expels this material, which discolors amniotic fluid to the well-known green color when motilin, an intestinal hormone, is released. The stimulus for the fetus to expel, or have a bowel movement, in the uterus is thought to be due to fetal stress. It is believed that one-fifth of all deliveries contain meconium. Whether or not this is correct, it is believed that the fetus is at risk under these circumstances. Meconium, whether thick or thin (diluted or concentrated), is damaging to fetal lungs if inhaled. It is also damaging to fetal membranes and can penetrate the membrane layers in one hour. If able to penetrate the amniotic barrier, cells called macrophages can transport these acids to the umbilical cord and can cause umbilical-vessel constriction. Experiments have demonstrated that umbilical arteries will be affected by meconium by stimulating the circular smooth muscle to tighten, thus closing the vessel off. This effect is observed to leave evidence of tissue damage as well as possible fetal circulation disturbances. Because meconium has the potential to lead to fetal compromise, it seems reasonable to avoid it. It is also possible that cord compression can cause the release of meconium by stimulating the release of motilin, creating additional cord-vessel constriction and blood flow interruption. This argues for close monitoring of fetuses with cord entanglement. The presence of meconium at birth does not mean or ensure that fetal damage has occurred. According to Dr. Naeye's study of the Collaborative Project, only 0.2% of the meconium-stained amniotic fluids examined were attributable to birth asphyxial disorders. However, Dr. Naeye stated: "After all of the antecedent risk factors had been taken into account, meconium in the amniotic fluid had only one unfavorable pregnancy outcome, the presence of neurological abnormalities at seven years of age. These neurologic abnormalities were of three types: quadriplegic cerebral palsy, lesser motor disorders with associated severe mental retardation, and chronic seizure disorders. These neurologic abnormalities are likely to be the consequence of vasoconstrictive effects of the meconium." A management goal,

JASON H. COLLINS, MD, MSCR

therefore, is to anticipate the fetus at risk and deliver it before a meconium accident. The timing may be difficult since it is believed that some fetuses can release meconium in small amounts and that it can be reabsorbed within twenty-four hours. There is debate about whether this is so, but it is known that the older the fetus, the more likely the occurrence. Fetuses are currently allowed to reach what is termed postmaturity. Yet fetuses older than a gestational age of forty-two weeks are considered postdates and are at risk of meconium. A management approach would be to consider any fetus with cord entanglement by its due date of forty weeks needs to be delivered. Doing so may avoid meconium in these infants as well as reducing stress factors to an already stressed state. In the Perinatal Umbilical Cord Project (PUCP), over one thousand fetuses have been screened, and no fetuses with obvious cord problems are delivered past forty weeks. None of these fetuses had meconium at delivery, suggesting that meconium is avoidable.

Ten percent of deliveries in the United States are associated with meconium. At least 1% have meconium complications. Fetuses prenatally diagnosed with umbilical cord complications should be aggressively managed to avoid meconium, and delivery should occur by forty weeks. Unless this issue is proven unimportant by future scientific studies, assuming that meconium is not dangerous seems risky. To date, no such study has been done. Managing a fetus identified with an umbilical cord risk eventually requires a decision to deliver the baby. Reaching that decision can be difficult, especially where the fetus is early. Prior to the delivery date, a series of evaluations is necessary to document the physiological state of the fetus. The avoidance of a premature delivery is the concern of the obstetrician or caregiver. Collecting information on how to decide when to deliver a compromised fetus sometimes depends on information derived within the hospital. The fetus can be studied in more detail and its movements assessed with ultrasound. For example, its amniotic fluid can be measured to look for decreased urine output. If the fetus is not making urine, it could suggest it is weak and, therefore, ready to deliver even though it is not in labor. The fetus's blood pressure can be indirectly checked with color Doppler flow measurements. Its average heart rate and reactions to induced contractions (oxytocin stress test) can be assessed. If it is abnormal, delivery can be initiated. Tools are available to manage umbilical cord-related fetal changes. Ultrasound, fetal monitoring, and fetal movement counts are all now available to evaluate fetal health. Currently, no prenatal blood test can be simply performed. Some tests can remove blood from the fetus by amniocentesis and indicate if delivery is necessary. These tests are risky and may themselves cause labor and delivery. Two tests are interesting to discuss. One is called a blood gas; the other is called erythropoietin. A blood gas is an absolute measurement of the fetal well-being. The fetus's oxygen level, pH level, and related chemistries such as base excess can be quickly determined. A needle must be used to remove blood from the umbilical vein, requiring transabdominal/uterine penetration. If the blood shows acidosis (a low pH), it suggests the fetus is in need of delivery. A more recently developed test that measures fetal reaction to oxygen levels is erythropoietin, a hormone specific to red blood cell production. Preliminary tests suggest that an elevated erythropoietin level means the fetus needs oxygen and should be delivered if the level is sustained. Erythropoietin may also play a role in protecting neurologic tissue as it has been identified in the brain. Newborns with increased red blood cell production may show changes in the blood count test. Nucleated red blood cells appear as a result of the increased erythropoietin stimulus. These are immature cells, and many appearing on a test suggest a closer look at the fetus. None of these tests individually can decide whether a fetus should be prematurely removed from the uterus. Taken together, they form a solid base from which clinical judgment still must decide intervention based on experience. Management of newborns with cord-accident-related births goes beyond labor. Several tests are important to consider if a compromised fetus is delivered. A third step to consider is a premature infant that is showing signs of stress from an umbilical cord problem. Situations such as monoamniotic twins have been managed where betamethasone was administered by thirty-one weeks. This was done to mature the fetal lungs in the event of early delivery after thirty-two weeks. There are now several examples published where this was done. A case study of a single fetus with a double nuchal cord and true knot was managed this way and is presented at the end of this book.

Morbidity—Other Effects

Nuchal-cord births have been observed to be predisposed to anemia. Not all nuchal-cord births are the same, but tight nuchal cords seem predisposed to producing anemia in the newborn. In one study, 18.5% of nuchal cords were anemic. The National Collaborative Perinatal Project defined perinatal anemia as a capillary hematocrit

JASON H. COLLINS, MD, MSCR

of less than 40% Hgb < 13.2 g/1 Hct < 39.1%. The information derived from this study suggests the need for hemoglobin and hematocrit determinations on all neonates who have nuchal cord [complications]. If symptomatic at delivery, hematologic evaluation should be done promptly and the neonate examined for evidence of hypovolemia and hypotension. If asymptomatic, hemoglobin and hematocrit determinations should be done before discharge from the nursery in order to identify those neonates who are anemic.

Angela J. Shepherd
Department of Pediatrics
University of Texas, Galveston
AJDC Vol. 139, 1/1985 pg. 71

Nuchal-cord deliveries may also cause loss of fetal blood volume that, if greater than 20%, will induce hypovolemic shock. This is a condition where the fetus has lost too much blood. Observations have been reported where blood transfusions were necessary to correct this emergency. The clinical picture is different from lack of oxygen in that blood volume is missing but oxygen levels are normal. The newborn is usually characteristically pale, tachycardiac with irregular respirations, and weak with a low blood pressure. This physiologic state is caused by decreased perfusion of tissue rather than an absence of oxygen and nutrients. The metabolic activity of the tissues remains static, so the chemical activity has nowhere to go—like a stagnant pond. Byproducts, therefore, have no place to go, and oxygen, although available, cannot enter the cell. The result is a buildup of waste products and carbon dioxide that results in cellular acidosis. This dangerous state can cause death if not corrected. Once discovered, hypovolemia is quickly treated with fluids, plasma, and blood transfusion. These events are not common but do happen. Indeed, knowing that the potential for morbidity exists can be enough to quickly recognize this clinical emergency. Newborns with cord problems should be reviewed for morbidity. Blood also contains cells that react to tissue damage called white blood cells (WBC). Many types of white blood cells are called by various names, depending on the cell purpose. A polymorphonuclear leukocyte (WBC/PMN) is a cell very important in protecting tissues from bacteria and other invaders. It is also important in reacting to tissue that has been damaged by changes in blood flow. Tissues that line blood vessels such as umbilical arteries and veins are called endothelial cells and, under high microscopic magnification, look like ceramic tiles. These cells contain chemicals that, when released, can react with PMNs and incur damage. These reactions over time can affect the smaller vessels of the placenta or elsewhere and eventually contribute to organ dysfunction. Not only does the fetus react as a whole to cord compression and as a biologic agent on a cellular level, but it also reacts on a molecular level. A rapidly emerging field in the medical sciences is one of molecular research. It is the step up from genetics and the step below cellular activity, but all are interrelated.

A possible marker for tissue damage is another WBC called a lymphocyte. Recent research by Dr. Naeye suggests that compromised fetuses that develop neurologic injury enough to cause cerebral palsy have changes in their lymphocyte counts. When reviewing records of a group of CP infants, lymphocyte counts of greater than ten thousand were noted. These elevations did not occur in any less severe circumstances and did not recur. The changes seem important in determining when neurologic injury took place. The timing of stillbirth will be discussed based on the appearance of the infant. These concepts of forensic studies are important if scientists are going to understand how umbilical cord accidents affect the fetus over time. With more multidimensional genetic markers and factors being uncovered, a better understanding of fetal death will emerge. What lies in the future is speculative, but now a solution is possible.

How Will Future Umbilical Cord-Complicated Pregnancies Be Managed?

The initial step is to visualize the baby. Mothers who have experienced a stillbirth should be studied with multiple ultrasounds during the subsequent pregnancy. Why? At the very least—to put them at ease. There is no unnecessary ultrasound in this group of patients. Very soon, 3-D printers will be able to translate the image into a physical product that can be held by the mother.

Nonstress test: "Our results suggest that the non-stress test should be used as the primary test for antepartum detection of fetal acidosis because it has the highest sensitivity; in addition, it is simple and easy to perform." (Vintzileos 1991)

JASON H. COLLINS, MD, MSCR

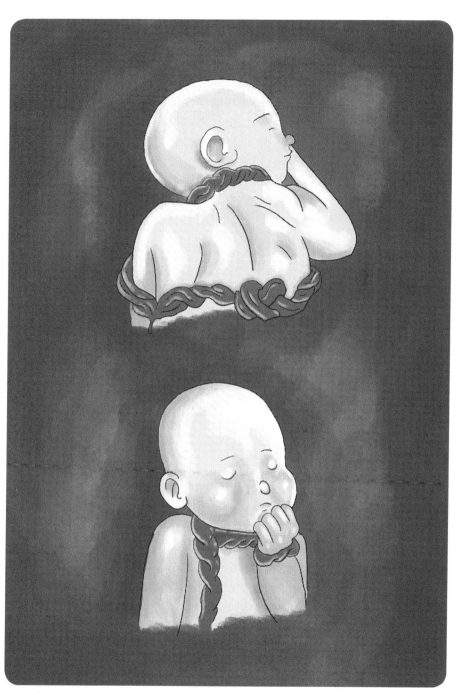

Managing UCA

CHAPTER SIX

The Future of Umbilical Cord Research

The goals of prenatal research must be to prevent cerebral palsy, to improve our understanding of prematurity, to give every baby its right to a sound body and mind when she or he is born, and perhaps one day make the NICU as obsolete as the iron lung [for polio].
—Peter W. Nathanielsz, MD, PhD, ScD
Ithaca, New York 1995

Where there is no vision, the people perish.
—Proverbs 29:18a KJV

What can be expected in the future of research into umbilical cord complications? To conduct the research, resources must be obtained to pay for the sophisticated technologies and supplies needed. Trained personnel such as nurse-midwives, medical statisticians, obstetricians, pathologists, and engineers will be needed, as well as competitive salaries. A review by the Institute of Medicine published in 1992 states that obstetrics and gynecology lack supporters in government research agencies. In its survey, it is estimated that six to eight physicians/scientists each year are recipients of major training support. Only 9 out of 250 departments of obstetrics and gynecology nationally received more than $2 million in federal funds in 1990. On one federal advisory committee, it was noted that there was a scarcity of obstetrics and gynecology representation even though a major source of hospital admissions to most acute-care hospitals is from ob/gyn. Overall, the share of research funds from federal sources going to departments of obstetrics and gynecology has remained at a steady 1.5%. Given adequate funding, the solution to umbilical cord complications is reachable. It appears possible that one solution to cord entanglement is to reach into the uterus and reverse it.

Today, Dr. Michael Harrison at the University of California, San Francisco, enters the uterus as early as twenty-four weeks' gestational age to repair holes in fetal diaphragms. This deadly defect, which occurs in about 1 of every 2,200 births, has been successfully treated this way.

Surgical manipulation of the uterus and fetus is highly complex and very risky. The demonstration that it can be done is equivalent to the Wright Brothers' first flight. The steps necessary to surgically repair diaphragmatic hernias are more involved than the steps it would take to untangle a fetus identified at risk, an event that may be many times more common than 1/2,200 for diaphragmatic hernia or 1/600 for mongolism risk. Every umbilical cord abnormality places the fetus at risk for stillbirth. This may be a 1/500 risk. Fetal harm without stillbirth may be 1/50 risk and unrecognized. Entering the uterus with an endoscope smaller than the diameter of a pencil is possible. By comparison to a uterine incision, the endoscope is significantly smaller. It essentially avoids trauma. Over the last decade, this experiment has been performed in animals and humans with success. This suggests that a fetus imaged with 3-D ultrasound and diagnosed with entanglement at twenty-four weeks can be identified. Fetal heart rate changes compatible with cord compression can be visually evaluated and a fetus at risk for complications followed. Today, needles are used to sample the umbilical cord for blood in infants with stress and illnesses. These invasive procedures are successful and proven to save fetuses' lives. A hook wire is inserted into the uterus to manipulate the cord. Several recent reports have used small-gauge devices to manipulate the cord, puncture it, and suture it. One report described the use of this technique to obstruct the cord of a dead twin who was taking blood flow from a live twin. All these efforts taken together say that entering the uterus with several small-diameter devices to visualize the fetus, identify the cord, remove the entanglement, and leave the fetus to heal and grow in the uterus is possible today. Reports from the Netherlands have demonstrated successful visualization of the fetus with an endoscope in monkeys, which does not disturb the mother or create premature labor. To accomplish the goal of fetal surgery for cord entanglement, funds are needed to design the equipment and to work with an established animal-model laboratory with trained technicians and certification. To purchase a research monkey for study and its necessary support costs at least $2,000 per monkey. This type of research is absolutely necessary to demonstrate to governmental authorities such as the Food and Drug Administration that these surgical techniques are safe and effective and can avoid stillbirth. Without this documentation, approval of these techniques will not take place.

Another approach being evaluated by the Pregnancy Institute uses fetal heart rate monitoring. Currently being studied is a surveillance approach that depends on telemetry (remote telephone monitoring). Selected patients with cord-entangled fetuses are equipped with special monitors at home. These home fetal heart rate monitors are used by the mother to record fetal heart rate strips for telephone transmission. At prescheduled times, the monitoring episodes are watched in real time by the physician at home. This allows the patient to be home and allows the physician to choose a convenient time. Surveillance with telemetry-based fetal heart rate monitoring is done every night until delivery, usually thirty-six to forty weeks. It has been done as early as twenty-eight weeks for two months straight. This clinical trial, as of this writing, has home monitored over one hundred patients with previous loss due to UCA. These patients are located across the United States and overseas.

> Stillbirth In non-malformed babies of birth weight greater than or equal to 2.51 kg. these babies are apparently well equipped to survive until the terminal event [normal but dead] and on the basis of this study there is likely to be a high degree of avoidability to their deaths. (Kirkup 1990)

Statistical understanding of umbilical cord-related stillbirths is inaccurate at best. Future efforts to more accurately depict events leading to stillbirth are needed. Publications from New Delhi, Norway, China, Scotland, Germany, Britain, and the United States cannot accurately determine how many antenatal or neonatal deaths are due to the umbilical cord. Because of inaccurate reporting by death certificates state by state, the National Center for Health Statistics cannot determine the extent of this mortality. Fetal harm (morbidity) is completely unknown and unavailable. One Chinese study suggested morbidity consisted of neurologic damage and neonatal deaths. What worldwide statistics exists is largely based on labor and delivery events and not prenatal events. One study reviewed perinatal deaths in normal infants and related lack of antenatal care by twenty weeks as an important risk factor. In 30% of deaths, there was an avoidable factor. In 61% of these cases, intrapartum management appeared to be an important factor. The most important aspect of management was recognition of fetal heart rate monitoring abnormalities.

In *Life* magazine, July 1969, Dr. Edward Hon is shown reading a fetal heart rate pattern recording from a fetal monitor he invented. The recording showed repeat fetal heart decelerations. An image of the delivered infant (breech delivery) was shown with of a single tight nuchal cord.

> Abnormal Fetal Heart Rate Patterns may be present for many minutes before actual fetal death. Changes in fetal heart rates associated with umbilical cord compression may be progressive over many minutes and hence useful . . . . Therefore, many of the avoidable factors detected related to the recognition of probable fetal distress by fetal heart rate monitoring these heart rate abnormalities arose 3 hours before death and did not resolve or remit but went unattended. (Hon 1975)

Estimating the time of death in stillborns is important in order to understand factors causing death. What events lead to the death of a fetus especially when the supply line is involved? In normal no-risk (no illness) pregnancies, this insight would be invaluable.

> A large review of cord related stillbirths needs to be done to determine the timing of death. Is it random, circadian, nightly, daily during maternal activity, rest, after meals, etc.? Here again there had been recognition of life within 4 days of delivery indicating that the fatal compression occurred with the advent of labor . . . . The mother had been uneasy about diminished foetal movements although the foetal heart was still distinctly heard; then within 2 days, the foetal heart disappeared. (Corkill 1961)

Some insights about the timing of death may be discoloration of the umbilical stump; desquamation (loss of skin) of the face, abdomen, or back; brown skin discoloration; and mummification. These changes correspond to six, twelve, twenty-four hours or to great changes from death to delivery. Reviewing stillbirths for these changes may help pinpoint time of death and fetal symptoms perceived by the mother.

Numerous examples have been published describing isolated case reports of maternal symptoms related to the cord mechanism involved. Reports include statements such as pulling sensations from the cord insertion site to great movements of the fetus as it changes position, or a stick on a picket fence, as the abdomen of the mother is stimulated with fetal repositioning. Fetal jerking movements and hiccups are not uncommon complaints with nuchal cords and knots. Rolling movements are detected by the mother. Even seizures have been described. The most important symptom is decreased fetal movement, sometimes days before death. We continue to tell patients that the fetus should not slow down toward term. The mother needs to be aware of fetal behavior. Patients can feel what the fetus is telling them. Every symptom and subtle sign should be used to suspect fetal compromise.

In European countries, intrauterine fetal death (IUFD) is responsible for more than half of the perinatal mortality rate. The intrauterine fetal death rate reflects the complete failure of pregnancy surveillance and antenatal care. Therefore, the development of specific strategies in order to further reduce stillbirths becomes more and more important. More than one-third of stillbirths reported in Europe seemed predictable and avoidable by appropriate management after a positive fetal surveillance test. More than 50% of the stillbirths occurred after the thirty-fourth week of gestation, when any infant has a nearly 100% chance to survive with modern pediatric care. At the same time, a marked decrease in the number of antenatal visits and quality of antenatal surveillance can be observed in cases of antepartum stillbirth. It should be concluded that antenatal surveillance has to be performed more intensively, especially in the last trimester.

> Intrauterine fetal death is the worst result of antenatal care for the obstetrician and creates tremendous grief with parents in the knowledge that they have lost an infant with full potentials for later life. (Scheider 1994)

Two types of deaths seem to be related to cord complications: sudden death, such as with cord rupture, hematoma, prolapse, and maybe entanglement;

JASON H. COLLINS, MD, MSCR

and slow death, such as with nuchal cords, knots, torsion, and body loops. There are early deaths and late deaths, which may have different patterns.

Management of patients facing this potential harm will require different strategies. Noninvasive approaches will use ultrasonography to discern the fetus at risk. Future evolution of techniques using chemical factors from the maternal blood may be useful in following that specific fetus. Detecting fetal chemical changes from the maternal blood sample may allow the evaluation of a slowly dying fetus and the decision to intervene with delivery if late or to intervene with manipulation of the fetus if early.

One older manipulation is external version. With computer assistance, knowing that the nuchal cord is entangled right to left, the fetus might be manipulated to unwind the loop. This is done by using one's hands on the pregnant abdomen and maneuvering the fetus around head to toe. These potential management techniques will have to be tried to determine their feasibility. To imagine this maneuver, compare it to the game of 3-D movements inside a round frame. Like the game, the procedure could be used to slowly rotate the mother to induce countermovements in the fetus, thus untangling it. Although this may seem far-fetched, with computer guidance and imaging, it may be possible. Another possible insight may be derived from NASA's Ames Research Center. NASA and specialists from the University of San Francisco's Fetal Treatment Center are developing devices that would be placed inside the uterus with the fetus. These devices would measure fetal vital signs. The intrauterine space becomes a tailored NICU. The biotransmitters send vital information by radio signal to be evaluated by computers outside the fetus. Already in existence is a thermometer capsule that is swallowed by astronauts to measure core body temperature. NASA codeveloped this capsule that sends constant temperature readings to a monitor by radio signal. The ability to continuously know fetal blood pressure, heart rate, EKG patterns, and oxygen/pH status will be important. Ultimately, it will be necessary to know glucose/lactic acid/catecholamine/erythropoietin and cortisol/ACTH levels. These chemistries provide insights into the fetal condition and would assist in deciding the need for delivery. For instance, a cord-entangled fetus with decreased movement, low oxygen levels, and elevated erythropoietin might need delivery. Current fetal blood tests attempting to determine time of injury only determine damage already done. These tests include measuring fetal lymphocyte counts over time. In the future, it may be possible to detect early changes as the damage is beginning and rescue the fetus before irreparable harm occurs.

Umbilical cord complications can be solved just as polio was solved. It is important to do so because the fetuses are normal. They are not defective, malformed, or irreparably injured. What is required is support to create the solutions. The solutions are at hand.

> At present, we can offer no single solution to the problem of umbilical cord complications which remains probably the most important cause of fetal depression at birth. (Bruce 1978)

> By means of a model similar to that of Clapp, et al we have reported evidence of an increase in free oxygen radicals as possible causal factor in cerebral lesion. These observations [of umbilical cord compression/blood flow reduction] should alert physicians to pursue more investigative studies on the potentially ominous FHR pattern in relation to the long term outcome of the infants, particularly that of neurologic performance. (Murata and Quilligan 1994)

Case Studies

(I) A Difficult Case for Prevention
A Combination Umbilical Cord Accident

This term pregnancy in a twenty-eight-year-old G3 P1 AB1 was uneventful until one weekend before the due date. Fetal movement ceased after a day-long fishing trip. Evaluation on labor and delivery indicated a fetal demise. Spontaneous vaginal delivery revealed a stillborn male fetus (7½ lb) with three nuchal cords, a shoulder loop-body loop, a two-vessel cord, straight architecture, and a true knot. In addition to these findings was a cord length of 100 cm and marginal placental insertion. Which abnormality caused death is disputed in the medical literature. When and how these fetuses die are difficult to document. Whether diet plays a role or maternal activity changes uterine physiology are unclear. The Perinatal Umbilical Cord Project (PUCP) seeks to address the problem of umbilical cord accidents.

JASON H. COLLINS, MD, MSCR

(II) Time of Death:
Nuchal Cord Type B and Clinical Clues

A thirty-year-old white female G1 P0 was doing well prenatally up until twenty-eight weeks when the fetus was noted to be breech turned from vertex. A single nuchal cord was diagnosed, and fetal heart rate changes were in normal range. Reexam at thirty weeks confirmed a breech lie with a NCX1 and normal FHR. A scheduled return in two weeks and expected repositioning of the fetus to vertex was preempted by stillbirth two days before the revisit. Saturday night, the patient noted fetal movement of normal strength and duration at 10:00 p.m. The fetus was breech and did not exhibit jerking movements or hiccups, suggesting no stress during the breech lie. Awakening at 7:00 a.m. on Monday morning, no movement was felt as expected. An office visit confirmed fetal demise, and an ultrasound showed a triple nuchal cord and a vertex lie. At delivery, a normal male (6 lb) had a triple NCX3 with a type B NCX1 (see text). Also seen was a marginal cord insertion into the placenta. Microscopic exam of the placenta showed chorangiosis (a placental change associated with asphyxia). The Perinatal Umbilical Cord Project (PUCP) has observed there are two types of nuchal cords (A and B) and that these stillbirths may occur at night during sleep.

(III) Fetal Heart Rate Changes:
Warning Signs of Cord Compression

Over one thousand pregnancy cases and counting have been reviewed for cord complications in the Perinatal Umbilical Cord Project. What has repeated itself over and over are the fetal heart rate patterns associated with cord compression. Depending on the degree of compression, duration, intermittency, and gestational age of the fetus, fetal heart rate responses tell us a lot about this event prior to labor. Three cases briefly described here suggest a variety of presentations.

Case KD
A thirty-year-old G3 P2 with normal deliveries previously. This fetus developed a shoulder loop and fetal heart rate changes prior to labor. Subsequent resolution of the shoulder loop occurred during a next-day OCT. Delivery was uneventful, but the newborn had a persistent ductus

arteriosus, and the placental exam showed chorangiosis, a pathology of placental stress. At five years old, the young girl is developing normally.

Case TR
A thirty-five-year-old G4 P3 developed an arrhythmia during labor. An intermittent arrhythmia was noticed prenatally. As labor progressed, the arrhythmia became more pronounced. Eventually the FHR became nonreassuring, causing a C-section. A posterior placenta with marginal/sacral umbilical insertion was present. The newborn EKG was abnormal for two hours. Cause unknown.

Case MB
A twenty-seven-year-old G1 P0 at term with a prenatally diagnosed nuchal cord X1 progressed to 6 cm, +1 station when sudden bradycardia developed. An emergency C-section was necessary to relieve the umbilical cord compression and developing metabolic acidosis. Note the developing arrhythmia and increasing frequency prior to delivery. A similar physiology may be the event occurring prenatally that leads to stillbirth of similar cases.

(IV) Umbilical Cord Risk Managed After a Previous Cord Accident

Case MS
A twenty-seven-year-old G2 P0 SB1 had a previous stillbirth associated with a double nuchal cord. Her subsequent pregnancy was monitored with frequent ultrasounds and FHR monitoring. At twenty-eight weeks, a double nuchal cord was seen on ultrasound. At thirty-two weeks, a true knot was verified. Delivery by thirty-six weeks confirmed a double nuchal cord with true knot. The patient correctly recognized decreased fetal movement and changes in the fetal heart rate (on home monitoring).

(IV) Umbilical Cord Risk Managed After a Previous
Cord Accident with Subsequent Morbidity TF

A twenty-eight-year-old G3 P1 SB1 was being monitored for repeat cord risk. Her previous stillbirth was due to a double nuchal cord and triple knot at thirty-six weeks. During the third pregnancy, a nuchal cord was diagnosed by thirty-two weeks and followed to thirty-six weeks, where decreased fetal movement and fetal heart rate variables prompted delivery. At forty-eight hours, the infant developed persistent pulmonary hypertension and required NICU care and oscillator support for one week. At six months, the newborn was well. Cord compression may be associated with pulmonary hypoxia due to shunts delivering blood flow to the adrenal gland, heart, and brain. Animal-model studies have suggested this connection. Recent computer cord-blood-flow models also suggest loss of pulmonary blood flow during fetal stress, hypotension, and low cord flow. Pulmonary injury may not be uncommon.

(VI) Umbilical Cord Torsion, a Not Uncommon Occurrence in Newborns

Umbilical cord torsion is usually not diagnosed in a live born. Ten percent of deliveries may have uncomplicated torsion. Torsion can coexist with constriction, a different pathology altogether. Amniotic bands may also be present with both the former pathologies. *No* published stillbirth study has included umbilical cord torsion in its database, which brings the results into question.

The following publication describes two cases of repeat UCA in the same mom. The explanation is that the fetal reflexes that lead to entanglement can recur under the same reproductive conditions. Patients have reported as many as four to five births each with nuchal cord, knots, and torsion. UCA events are not rare; they can repeat in the same mom and family (such as long cords) and can repeat similar developmental characteristics.

Multiple tight coils of funis with repeated fetal death.

by MM. H. Vermelin and J. Richon
"Multiples circulaires serrés avec mort foetale"
Société d'obstétrique et de gynécoogie de Nancy
1950
(Traduced from French by Laura Adam)
10/15/2009

Multiples tight coils of funis with repeated fetal deaths
Let us describe you two observations:

Observation 1.—Ms. A . . . , 29 years old, mother of two daughters aged of 10 and 2 years old, became pregnant in January 1950. She was supposed to give birth by the end of October.

The 10th of October, she feels the first contractions and enters in the maternity hospital. After a rapid 3 hours labor, she ejects a 3.400 kg boy. His head is freeing up with difficulties and remains locked at the vulva. We hardly lower the occiput and notice that there exists, at the neck emplacement, three tight coils of funis, so tight that the umbilical cord has a reduced volume, forming a real whitish lace. After rapidly cutting the cord, we notice that the baby's neck is cut by the coils and that the skin is snatched at certain sites. The child hasn't any heart beats anymore: he is pale and cannot be resuscitated. The cord's length was 44 cm. This woman gets pregnant two years after. The childbirth was planned for the last days of June. The 1st of July, when she enters in the maternity hospital, the head is high but applies conformably to the [DS???]. The cervix is dilated to 3 cm. Two hours later, the dilatation is complete. The head is at the medium part. Because of the previous incidents, we check very regularly the fetal heart after each contraction. Foetus heart beats are goods. As soon as the urge to eject the baby arrives, beats remain very slow after each contraction and we decide to finish with an application of forceps in [GT ???], at the medium part of the excavation. With some difficulties, we bring the head at the lower part, and as in the first case, the enucleation of the head is difficult: we notice with astonishment, four coils of funis very tight, binding the neck of the foetus, that we promptly cut. We extract the baby: a 3.400 kg boy without any heart beat. The cord measured 50 cm.

Observation 2.—Ms. S . . . is 29 years old in 1951.

She gave birth in 1947 in the maternity hospital, in 1949 at home, and in 1951 at Charleville, two boys and a girl that grew up normally.

The 30th of April 1954, she delivers a 3.800 kg boy at home; he presents the start of a fetus sanguinolentus and has one very tight coil of funis.

Her fifth delivery takes place the 1st of March, 1956. At noon, when she enters at the maternity hospital, the dilatation was 4 cm—the amniotic sac was intact—fetal beats were irregular and muffled.

At 5pm, spontaneous split of the pouch: mushy pea liquid. The head was at the high part of the excavation in [G.P. ??]. Beats not sensed.

At 7pm, complete dilatation and ejection of a boy weighting 3.600kg in 10 minutes. There exists one tight coil that we cut using pliers. The baby is flabby but presents some heartbeats.

The baby dies in [word absolutely unknown, it sounds like "slightly raised from death"], a few minutes after, despite the usual cares.

If we look at the death toll of this sinister series of foetus deaths, one recent foetus sanguinolentus and three fetal death at ejection, we can only notice the presence of the danger of coiling of funis.

This danger is a constant threat and the fact that it is unpredictable makes it more serious.

At present, there is no investigation method to asses or declare null the existence of coils in the cord. Even if one day we can predict, before delivery, the presence of one or more coils, how many children are born with loose coils.

Too many considerations are involved: length of the cord, thickness of the cord, movement of the foetus, repetitive careful attempts of [version??] by external operations, which each of them or all of them, can create one or more coils.

The late engagement to the presentation due to the fact that the foetus is trussed by a short cord is not a possible criterion for tight coils above all for the multiparous.

The only solution for the obstetrician is to check the quality of the foetus heart beats, far from being an absolute solution. How many times beats are slowly and affected for a while during the ejection.

Proceeding to an emergency Caesarean section when we know there were previously a mortal foetal accident can appears as a legitimate advise, in condition that this caesarean is wittingly made, for an healthy foetus and not for a dying foetus on which anoxia would have already causes irreversible encephalo-meningal [???] lesions. And how many useless sections will be practice in those cases! At present, it seems that obstetrical trauma, cause of the fetal death by funic compression (cord prolapses and coils of funis) represent 1% of neonatal deaths. Canon, Guillem and Mayer evaluated in 1953 to 9% the risk of neonatal anoxia purely due to funic.

Anoxia caused by funic remains a heavy mortgage weighting on delivery and which doesn't seem to be definitively removed presently.

A recent e-mail tells the same story of repeat loss due to UCA.

From: Erica
To: haydel1@bellsouth.net;
Date: Tue, January 15, 2008 11:13:48 PM
Cc:

Subject: Dr. Collins, I have had two stillborn babies Dr. Collins, I am 27 years old. I read about you online and the research you are doing on stillborn babies. My first baby was stillborn at almost 35 weeks in August of 2006 and I recently lost my second baby at 30 weeks on December 18, 2007. We have no answers as to why this has happened twice. The doctors see nothing wrong with the cord, placenta, etc. Both baby girls have been born looking perfectly healthy and the first autopsy revealed nothing, we are still waiting on results for our 2nd baby's autopsy. I believe that they both passed away in the middle of the night because I felt each of them moving before I went to sleep and felt no movement the next day. My husband and I desperately want a healthy baby and are devestated that this nightmare has happened twice.

I appreciate your time.

Erica

Umbilical cord accidents can repeat in the same patient (mother). They can be identified with ultrasound, managed with fetal heart rate monitoring, and successfully delivered. No baby should be stillborn after thirty-six weeks due to a UCA. The solution requires intensive observation and identification of the fetus at risk for this silent complication. The following protocol can help prevent UCA.

JASON H. COLLINS, MD, MSCR

Protect your Pregnancy-Pregnancy Institute Protocol

Ultrasound Can Visualize the Umbilical Cord

10-12 weeks: a vaginal ultrasound to measure the crown-to-rump length of the baby.

18-20 weeks: anatomical description of the umbilical cord and its placental and fetal connections.

26-28 weeks: umbilical cord review documenting its position and characteristics.

30-32 weeks: umbilical cord review documenting its position and characteristics.

36-37 weeks: umbilical cord review noting the presence of cord entanglement, twisting, compression location near the rump or baby's head.

If an ultrasound review documents a finding, more frequent prenatal visits are needed. After twenty-six weeks, the baby has a good chance of survival if delivered early. If entanglement is noted on an ultrasound study, weekly ultrasounds will be needed. Fetal heart rate testing twice a week is needed. Babies can relieve entanglement and twisting. Those that cannot are vulnerable to problems that can be detected by fetal behavior monitoring and maternal awareness of the problem.

By twenty-six to twenty-eight weeks, the baby establishes its behavior patterns. A common pattern is for the baby to move at bedtime once the mother becomes supine. This event causes maternal blood flow shifts that the baby detects. It responds with reflex movement to reestablish its blood flow. This intrauterine reflex is a reliable sign of a healthy baby. If the baby moves a lot (hyperactivity) or moves less than normal, the mom should be evaluated on labor and delivery at that time. Taking these steps will be the best chance of achieving a live birth where UCA exists.

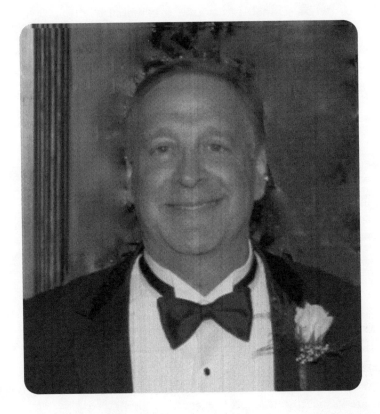

Dr. J. Collins is from New Orleans, Louisiana, and trained with Tulane Medical Center. He specializes in obstetrics and gynecology. He recently completed a master's degree in clinical research from Tulane Medical Center. He is the principal investigator for the PUCP (Perinatal Umbilical Cord Project). The study reviewed over one thousand no-risk pregnancies for UCA and is peer reviewed and published by the Royal College of Obstetrics and Gynecology.

RECOMMENDED READING

Amiel-Tison, Claudine and Ann Stewart, eds. *The Newborn Infant: One Brain for Life*. Published by the National Institute of Health and Medical Research. Paris, France. 1994.

"Ann Jillian's Miracle Baby—Delivery Room Drama" (with a triple nuchal cord discovered at C-section). *National Enquirer* (February 25, 1992).

Arvy, L. and G. Pillepi, eds. 1976. "Le Cordon Ombilical (Fonis Umbilicalis)." Ostermundigen, Switzerland.

Atlas, Jan, ed. 2010. *They Were Still Born*. (Amazon.com).

Benirschke, Kurt and Peter Kaufman. 1990. *Pathology of the Human Placenta*. 2nd ed. New York, New York: Springer-Verlag.

Birnholz, Jason C. 1990. "Ecologic Physiology of the Fetus, Ultrasonography of Supply-Line Deprivations Syndromes." Radiologic Clinics of North America 28 (1): 179.

Brier, B. The murder of Tutankhamon, Berkeley Books NY, 1999, 116-117

Bukowski, R. et al. 2011. "Causes of Death Among Stillbirths." *Journal of the American Medical Association* 306 (22): 2459-2468. doi:10.1001/jama.2011.1823.

Cabaniss, Miki L., ed. 1993. *Fetal Monitoring Interpretation*. Philadelphia, Pennsylvania: J. B. Lippincott Co.

Clark, SL. et. al. 2013 Intrapartum Management of Category II heart rate tracings: Towards Standardization of Care. American Journal of Obstetrics and Gynecology 209.

Clapp, James F., III et. al. 1988. "Brain Damage After Intermittent Partial Cord Occlusion in the Chronically Instrumented Fetal Lamb." *American Journal of Obstetrics and Gynecology* 159: 504.

Collins, J. H. 2002. "Umbilical Cord Accidents: Human Studies." *Semin Perinatol* 26 (1): 79-82.

Collins, J. H. 2012. BMC Pregnancy and Childbirth 12 (Suppl 1): A7. http://www.biomedcentral.com/1471-2393/12/S1/A7.

Collins, J. H. and C. L. Collins. Edited by J. Kingdom, E. Jauniaux, and S. O'Brien. "The Human Umbilical Cord." In *The Placenta: Basic Science and Clinical Practice* 2000: 319-329. Ch 26. London: RCOG Press.

Collins, J.H., C. L. Collins, and C. C. Collins. 2010. "Umbilical Cord Accidents." http://www.preginst.com/UmbilicalCordAccidents2.pdf.

Corkill, T. F. 1961. "The Infant's Vulnerable Life-Line." *Australian New Zealand Journal of Obstetrics and Gynecology* 1: 154.

De Hann, Harmen H. et. al. 1997. "Brief Repeated Umbilical Cord Occlusions Cause Sustained Cytotoxic Cerebral Edema and Focal Infarcts in Near-Term Fetal Lambs." *Pediatric Research* 41: 96.

Feinstein, Steven J. "Intrapartum Ultrasound Diagnosis of Nuchal Cord as a Decisive Factor in Management."

Harman, Christopher R., ed. 1995. *Invasive Fetal Testing and Treatment.* Winnipeg, Canada: Blackwell Scientific Publications. ISBN 0-86542-208-7.

Heifetz, S.A. Edited by S. H. Lewis and E. Perrin. "Pathology of the Umbilical Cord." In *Pathology of the Placenta.* 2nd ed. 1999: 1007-136. New York, New York: Churchill Livingstone.

Hon, Edward. 1969. "Watching the Unborn Inside the Womb: High Risk Mothers and the Graph that Raises Their Babies' Chances." *Life Magazine* (July 25) 63-66.

Kevin Kanty—"Death Before Life, An Account of Stillbirth due to Umbilical Cord Torsion." *Vogue* (May 1995) 93-96.

Kohner, Nancy and Alix Henley. 1995. *When a Baby Dies: The Experience of Late Miscarriage, Stillbirth, and Neonatal Death.* San Francisco, California: Harper Collins Publishers. ISBN 004-440-934-6.

Lee, ST, HON EH. Fetal hemodynamic response to umbilical cord compression. Obstet Gynecol 1963, 22: 553-562.

Mann, Leon. 1986. "Pregnancy Events and Brain Damage." *American Journal of Obstetrics and Gynecology* 155: 6.

Murata, Yuji et. al. 1994. "Variable Fetal Heart Rate Decelerations and Electrocortical Activities." *American Journal of Obstetrics and Gynecology* 170: 689.

Naeye, Richard L. 1992. *Disorders of the Placenta, Fetus, and Neonate: Diagnosis and Clinical Significance.* St. Louis, Missouri: Mosby Year Book.

Nathanielsz, Peter W. 1992. *Life Before Birth and a Time to be Born.* Ithaca, New York: Promethean Press.

Nelson, Karin B. and Jonas H. Ellenberg. *Antecedents of Cerebral Palsy.* National Institute of Neurological and Communicative Disorders and Stroke.

Nijhuis, J. G., ed. 1992. *Fetal Behaviour: Developmental and Perinatal Aspects.* Oxford, England: Oxford University Press.

Nilsson, Lennart. Text by Lars Hamberger. 1993. *A Child is Born.* New York: Bantam Doubleday Dell Publishing Group Inc. ISBN 0-440-50691-3.

Pfaffin, ed. 1994. *Annals of the New York Academy of Sciences* 736.

Reynolds, Samuel R. 1952. "The Umbilical Cord." *Scientific American* 187 (July): 70.

Ryan, W. D. et. al. "Placental Histologic Criteria for Diagnosis of Cord Accident: Sensitivity and Specificity." *Pediatric and Developmental Pathology* 2012 (15): 275-80. Department of Pathology University of San Diego, California.

Sadovsky, E. et. al. "Decreased Fetal Movements Associated with Umbilical Cord Complications." Israel. JMed Sci 1977 Mar; 13 (3): 295-8 ISR.

Simpson, Joe Leigh and Sherman Elias, eds. 1994. *Fetal Cells in Maternal Blood: Prospects for Noninvasive Prenatal Diagnosis.* New York, New York: New York Academy of Sciences.

Smotherman, William P. and Scott R. Robinson. 1988. *Behavior of the Fetus.* Caldwell, New Jersey: Telford Press.

Strong, Tom H. 1993. "Non-Coiled Umbilical Cord Vessels: A New Marker for the Fetus at Risk." *Obstetrics and Gynecology* 81: 409.

"Today's Latest Coo—Deborah Norville's Delivery" (which includes an umbilical cord knot). *People* (March 25, 1991) 67-73.

Torpin, Richard. 1974. *Reproduction in Man and His Ancestors for 700 Million Years.* McGowen Printing Company.

Townsend, Jessica, ed. 1992. *Strengthening Research in Academic Ob/Gyn Departments.* Washington, DC: National Academy Press.

Wilson, B. 2008. "Sonography of the Placenta and Umbilical Cord." *Radiologic Technology* 79 (4): 333-345S.

JASON H. COLLINS, MD, MSCR

INDEX

A

abnormalities
  cord, 14, 25, 41, 82
  fetal/placental, 50
  identifiable umbilical cord, 18, 39
  neurologic, 27-28, 84
  placental insertion/location, 83
  umbilical placental, 39
acid, lactic, 66
age, 40, 66-67, 71, 84
  gestational, 14, 27, 40-41, 43-44,
    47, 50-51, 73, 85, 91, 97
animal models, 59, 66-67, 69-71, 73, 75
animal research, 50, 68-69
anomalies, 9, 18, 26, 30-31, 39, 79
anoxia, 101
antenatal care, 93-94
antenatal surveillance, 94
arrhythmia, 66, 71, 98
arteries, 14, 19-21, 23, 25-26, 29,
    32-33, 35-36, 42, 46, 52, 82
  umbilical, 23, 25, 34-36, 49, 74-75,
    84, 87

B

baby, 10, 13, 18, 20, 31, 64, 79, 81,
    85, 88, 90, 92, 100-103, 107
  healthy, 102-3
  stillborn, 102
birth, 13, 15, 18, 21, 25, 32-33, 36, 40,
    49, 52-53, 58-59, 61-64, 73-74,
    81, 84, 91, 96, 99-100, 107

premature, 14, 33
birth weight, 92
blood, 25, 34-36, 67, 74-75, 86-87,
    91, 108
blood flow, 14, 24-25, 27, 29-30, 32,
    34, 36, 40-41, 43, 54, 60, 64-66,
    70-77, 82, 87, 91, 99, 103
  placental, 70, 76
blood flow interruption, 71, 84
blood gas, 86
blood loss, 36, 67, 74-75
blood pressure, 43, 64-65
  fetal, 22, 36, 70, 72, 85, 95
blood transfusions, 87
blood vessels, 34-36, 71, 87
brain, 60, 65-66, 70-73, 86, 99, 105
breech, 28, 45, 97

C

carbon dioxide, 66, 87
cells, 31, 66, 72-74, 84, 87-88
  stem, 19, 21
cerebral palsy, 15, 18, 31, 72, 80, 90,
    107
cervix, 31, 40, 42-43, 100
chemicals, 62, 65, 72, 74, 88
chemistries, 25, 36, 65, 70, 86, 95
chorangiosis, 76-77
circulation, 35-36, 46, 72
  cord, 46
clots, 34
coils, 24, 81, 100-101

compression, 27, 33, 40, 42, 49, 60,
    64-65, 70
constriction, 25, 29-30, 32, 35, 42,
    53, 75, 99
contractions, 60, 72, 100
cord, 13-14, 19-20, 22-29, 31-34, 36,
    40-55, 57, 64-65, 67, 71-72, 75,
    80-82, 91, 93, 100-102, 108
  abnormal, 28
  defective, 67
  double, 26
  double nuchal, 37, 84, 86, 98
  entangled, 35, 80
  equine, 51
  four-vessel, 26, 30
  fused, 23
  helical, 33
  knotted, 54
  long, 21-23, 30, 42-43, 80, 82, 99
  normal, 20
  prolapsed, 40-41, 54, 67
  proximal, 19, 24
  short, 22, 28, 30-31, 42, 48, 52, 67,
      80, 101
  single umbilical artery, 32
  spiraled, 51
  torsioned, 47, 51
cord accidents, 45, 80, 83, 98, 108
cord architecture, 26, 47
cord attachment, 58
cord blockage, 43, 66
cord coilings, 44, 50, 52, 57, 81, 101
cord compression, 34, 40, 46, 49,
    54-55, 59-60, 64-66, 70-73, 76,
    83-84, 88, 91, 97, 99
  chronic, 73
  complete, 65, 71
  gradual, 55
  incomplete, 40
  infrequent, 59
  intermittent partial, 67

intermittent umbilical, 76
prenatal umbilical, 15
prolonged, 72
umbilical, 40, 56, 59, 70-73, 77, 93,
    98, 107
cord design, 29, 36, 46
cord insertion, 33
  abnormal, 33
  abnormal placental, 18, 59
  furcate, 33
  marginal, 97
cord length, 22-24, 26-28, 31, 36,
    41-42, 51, 82, 96
  abnormal, 21
  decreased, 31
  multigravida, 22
  shorter, 23
cord-length effects, 42
cord rupture, 20, 33, 94
cord tension, 49
cord vessels, 32, 34, 48-49, 55, 75
C-section, 14, 31, 40, 42, 98, 105
cysts, 30, 33

D

death, 9, 13, 18-20, 41, 45-46, 49-50,
    52, 54, 76, 92-94, 96-97, 105, 107
  cord-related, 9, 15
  fetal, 14, 27, 45, 50, 53-54, 70, 88,
      93, 101
    intrauterine, 94
    term intrapartum, 45
  neonatal, 92-93, 101, 107
delivery, 18, 21-22, 24, 27, 29, 33-34,
    39, 41-42, 44, 46, 48-49, 52,
    54-55, 57, 67, 70, 73, 79-80, 82,
    84-87, 92-101, 103
  breech, 93
  early, 86
  immediate, 67, 70

normal, 97
nuchal-cord, 44, 86-87
premature, 85
vaginal, 42, 60
dilatation, 100
disabilities, learning, 9, 15, 18, 80
disruption, 18, 29-30, 39-40, 42, 67
ductus venosus, 60, 65

E

edema, 28, 30, 33-34, 48, 71
embryo, 19, 25, 32, 61
endoscope, 91
entanglement, 21, 30, 41-43, 46, 91,
    94, 99, 103
  cord, 14, 28, 43, 46, 60, 77, 81,
    84-85, 91-92, 103
  fetal, 22, 43, 83
erythropoietin, 86

F

fetal behavior, 10, 34, 43, 49, 52,
    61-62, 83, 94
fetal compromise, 26, 28, 67, 84, 94
fetal distress, 33, 42, 44, 80, 93
fetal harm, 18, 30, 32-36, 40, 50, 77,
    80, 91-92
fetal heart rate monitoring, 11, 15, 57,
    92-93, 102
fetal heart rate patterns, 22, 97
fetal movements, 10, 22-23, 42, 46,
    54, 61, 63, 83, 85, 96
fetal senses, 62
fetus, 9-11, 14, 18-37, 39-47, 49,
    51-55, 57-66, 69-73, 75-77,
    80-88, 91, 93-97, 102, 105,
    107-8
  active, 27, 43, 45
  anencephalic, 60

breech-positioned, 28, 45
compromised, 10, 24, 83, 85-86, 88
cord-entangled, 55, 82, 92, 95
live-born, 15
stillborn, 44
stressed, 83
term, 28, 41
FHR (fetal heart rate), 15, 55, 70, 83,
    91, 93, 98, 103
fluid, amniotic, 27, 42-43, 62, 73, 75,
    84-85
funis, 99-101

G

ganglion, phrenic, 60
gland, adrenal, 72-73, 99
glucose, 61, 65-66, 72
glycogen, 65-66, 72
gynecology, 81-82, 90-91, 104-8

H

head, 40, 45, 63, 95, 100
heart, 19, 27, 32, 35, 65-66, 70-71,
    73, 99
  fetal, 24-25, 35-36, 42, 57, 65, 72,
    100
heart failure, 50-51
heart rate, 61, 65, 70-71, 95
helixes, 24, 51
  umbilical cord, 24, 52
hematoma, 34, 42, 47-49, 82, 94
  umbilical cord, 49
hemoglobin, 87
hernias, 28-29
hiccups, 59-60, 94, 97
HUVECs (human umbilical vein
    endothelial cells), 21
hypovolemia, 87
hypoxia, 26, 70, 72

I

infants, 11, 29, 32, 40, 45-47, 49, 60, 67, 80-82, 85, 88, 91, 94, 96, 99, 106
insertion, 22, 32-33, 47
  abnormal placental, 82
  low placental, 81
  marginal placental, 96
  membranous, 29, 33
intestines, 19

K

kidney, 26-27, 64-65, 70, 72-73, 76
knot formations, 45, 47
knots, 40, 46-47, 53-54, 82, 94-95, 99
  complex, 54
  true, 14, 22, 41, 47, 51, 53-54, 81, 86, 96, 98

L

labor, 22, 27-28, 30, 41-42, 44, 48-49, 57-59, 62, 67, 74, 79-82, 85-86, 93, 96-98, 103
  premature, 30, 33, 36, 91
LBWC (limb-body wall complexes), 22
life, 18, 26, 42, 58, 93-94, 105, 107
  extrauterine, 62
  fetal, 31, 45, 62, 72-73
  intrauterine, 51-52, 58, 60, 62
liver, 27, 32, 60, 65, 72-73
loops, 45-46, 52-54, 81, 95
  body, 14, 41, 46, 48, 54-55, 80, 95
  cord, 14, 54
  nuchal, 45, 47
  shoulder, 48, 80, 97
lordosis, 58
lungs, 66, 73
lymphocyte, 88

M

manipulation, 69, 95
meconium, 35, 62, 84-85
mitochondria, 72
morbidity, 15, 76, 86-87, 92
mother, 9, 15, 18, 21, 28, 43-44, 53, 57-59, 63, 70, 72-74, 76-77, 80, 83, 88, 91-95, 100, 102-3
motilin, 84
MRI (magnetic resonance imaging), 25, 58

N

neonates, 27, 87, 107
nerve, phrenic, 24, 60
newborns, 7, 28, 32-33, 59, 62-63, 86-87, 97, 99
nitric oxide, 74
nuchal cord formation, 45
nuchal cords, 14, 20, 41, 44-48, 53, 81, 86-87, 94-99, 106
  single, 97
  triple, 55, 97, 105
nutrition, 20, 27, 36

O

obstetricians, 9-10, 14, 28, 36, 39, 61, 81-82, 85, 90, 94, 101
obstetrics, 14, 26, 40, 48, 59, 69, 81-82, 90, 104-8
organs, 19, 29, 66, 72-74, 76
oxygen, 25-26, 35-36, 41, 64-67, 69-71, 74, 77, 86-87
oxygen deprivation, 69, 71
oxygen levels, 65, 86-87
  low, 76-77, 95

P

pathology, 45, 50, 58, 73, 98-99
physiology, 11, 27, 35, 44, 57, 61, 98
placenta, 9, 13, 19-21, 23-29, 31-33,
    35-36, 38, 42, 46, 48, 50, 58,
    63, 67, 70-72, 74-76, 79-80, 82,
    88, 97, 102, 105-7
  abnormal, 37
  normal, 20
  posterior, 98
position, 19, 22, 43, 51, 55, 57-58,
    61-65, 81-82, 94, 103
  fetal, 46, 53, 59, 63
  placental, 22, 25, 45, 52, 58
pregnancies, 21-23, 26-28, 34-35, 39,
    43-44, 50, 58-59, 79, 83, 88,
    93, 98
Pregnancy Institute, 9, 11, 15, 50, 92
prolapse, 40, 42, 94
  cord, 80, 101
PUCP (Perinatal Umbilical Cord
    Project), 15, 85, 96-97, 104

R

reflexes, 43, 55, 59-61, 63-64
  startle, 63-64
repositioning, 47, 51-52, 61, 64

S

separation, placental, 55, 67
shunts, 32, 73, 99
site
  placental implantation, 19
  placental insertion, 82
souffle, placental, 64
Stillbirth Collaborative Research
    Network, 18
stillbirth risk, 31-32

stillbirths, 13-14, 18-19, 23-26, 30,
    32, 34-36, 40-41, 47, 51, 54, 76,
    80, 88, 91-94, 97-98, 105, 107
  antepartum, 94
  cord-related, 11, 92
  fetal, 9, 33
  recurrent, 18
stillborns, 14, 49-50, 81, 93, 96, 102
strength, tensile, 20
stress, 51, 66, 72-74, 86, 91, 97
  fetal, 83-84, 99
SUA (single umbilical artery), 22-23,
    32, 41
system, vestibular, 55

T

teratomas, 34
thrombosis, 24, 34, 48, 50, 76
torque, 47, 51-52, 54
torsion, 18, 22, 47-48, 50-54, 57, 76,
    83, 95, 99
  cord-related, 50
  umbilical cord, 50, 99, 107
toxemia, 14, 31-32, 34
trisomy, 48
tumors, 28, 33-34
twins, 23, 26, 31, 40-41, 53
  monoamniotic, 40-41, 53, 86
twists, 24, 47, 50-52, 54

U

UCA (umbilical cord abnormalities),
    10, 14-15, 18, 20, 22-25, 30, 79,
    92, 99, 102-4
ultrasound, 10, 15, 23, 25, 43-45, 53,
    58-60, 63, 76, 81-83, 85, 88, 91,
    97-98, 102-3
  vaginal, 15, 103

umbilical cord, 11, 13-14, 17-37, 39-54, 58-60, 63-64, 70, 74-75, 79-82, 84, 91-92, 96, 100, 103, 108

abnormal, 30

absent, 42

accidents, 7, 9, 11, 14, 18, 50, 69, 80, 88, 96, 102, 106

complications, 15, 52, 76, 108

development, 20, 24, 32

four-vessel, 32

long, 22, 31, 42

normal, 24, 28

prolapsed, 40

rupture, 48, 67

short, 30-31, 42

thin, 82

vessels, 19, 26, 34, 48, 74-75

umbilical cord attachments, 24, 29

umbilical vein, 19, 21, 24-25, 30, 32-36, 42, 47, 49, 60, 75, 86

umbilicus, 19, 26, 29-31, 49

uterus, 11, 14, 20, 25, 33-34, 40, 42-43, 46, 54, 57-59, 61-63, 67, 70, 81, 84, 86, 91, 95

V

vasopressin, 66, 72

vertex, 45, 97

VI (Velamentous insertion), 25, 29-30, 48, 59, 99

W

WBC (white blood cells), 87-88

Wharton's jelly, 19-20, 27, 30-35, 49, 52

content, 20, 27

Made in the USA
Lexington, KY
03 December 2013